Breast Cancer Treatment...
the decisions are YOURS

By

Jean Macpherson Duffy

This book is a work of non-fiction. Names and places have been changed to protect the privacy of all individuals. The events and situations are true.

ISBN: 1-4107-3186-3 (e-book)
ISBN: 1-4107-3185-5 (Paperback)
ISBN: 1-4107-4458-2 (Dust Jacket)

This book is printed on acid free paper.

1stBooks - rev. 05/14/03

Dedication

This book is dedicated

To my husband
Gordon West Duffy
With unending love and great appreciation
for the
Support and encouragement not only during
The cancer experience, but also
For believing that I should
"push my envelope"
and express myself
in
writing

TABLE OF CONTENTS

FOREWORD

There are many resources available for the person diagnosed with cancer. Why would I add one more? I had a very small tumor, easily operable, and have a 90% survival rate. But, I have the desire to share all that I learned on my six-month medical journey.

Breast cancer is in a category by itself by the very nature of the cancer's location. I certainly re-discovered the extent our society is concerned with *breasts*. Every catalog that came to our house had a gorgeous young woman with full and rather exposed breasts leaping off the cover page. Health magazines are filled with articles and pictures about jogging bras and nursing bras and how to care for breasts during sports activities, pregnancy and nursing. Time magazine featured a cover and long article on breast cancer. And visit any magazine store and peruse the men's section - breasts are very prominent everywhere.

So breast cancer treatment of any kind will, by virtue of its location, make you come to terms with your own breasts and thus your own sexuality. If I felt that this was true for me as a postmenopausal woman, I can only imagine it to be magnified for a younger woman. So many treatment options, so many decisions, but ultimately you must live with your changed body!

Remembering that it is YOUR body sounds so simple, but this fact gets lost once you start down the path toward medical care. Even though I am a nurse and was a state legislator writing laws about health care, I still experienced fear, confusion, frustration and tears. I hope that my readers will not be like a woman I read about recently in a "Letter to the Editor" of a popular health magazine. She wrote, "I am taking Tamoxifen, *which I am required to do to keep my oncologist...."*

Health care professionals included in my story have fictitious names and are presented as a composite of the many attitudes that I encountered. The bottom line is this: ask questions, ask more questions, change doctors or disagree with the health care profession if need be. This is your life and you must be in the driver's seat. You can still live happily every after. I have, and you can too.

Acknowledgements

When I was keeping a journal during my breast cancer experience, I was never sure that I would do anything with it once the treatments were finished. I decided to write a few pages to see whether or not I felt that I had a story to tell. The teacher in me desperately wanted to share with other women the need to be their own best advocate. And so I started to write.

I asked several friends to read what I had written. If they had been less than encouraging, I never would have continued. And therefore I have Reva Basch, Rob Elder, Rob Diefenbach, and Alice Dienfenbach to thank for providing the impetus to go on. They not only read the content, but also spent time going over the drafts and offering great suggestions.

I asked my women friends to share their experiences with hormones and hormone replacement therapy. I thank the women in my Circle, and the women in the So-no-men for being so willing to share.

I thank the Gingers with whom I tap danced for ten years for encouraging me to finish the book and not to give up when I became tired.

I thank my grown children for acknowledging that I could try writing as a new pursuit even though "writer" is a title they never before associated with me. Their love and support during the actual period from diagnosis through radiation made recovery much easier.

The hero of my story is the unsung hero of the medical team - the pathologist. Through the span of thirteen years from one diagnosis to another, Dr Michael Lagios has always been honest and practical in his advice.

Thanks also to my Nurse Practitioner, Lois Falk, for hearing my plea and respecting my needs.

A huge feeling of gratitude and unending thanks to my editor, Frances DeNisco. Besides holding a full time job and mothering two pre-school children, she made time for this manuscript. Frances forced me, with her pointed pencil, to communicate in a less formal and more compassionate manner.

To my daughter, Lorna Moorhead, a published writer, who edited the back page photo -- thank you for your fine artistic strokes..

And of course I wish to acknowledge my old friend Grant Campbell who offered suggestions and encouragement about publishing. Thanks to George Rathmell who did the same.

I thank all of those I met on this journey with breast cancer for without them there would be no message to communicate to others facing this diagnosis.

And finally to my wonderful husband, Gordon. Without his support I would never have taken the time nor endured the discipline necessary to complete this book

CHAPTER I
HOW IT ALL STARTED

So, it was to be a routine mammogram. My husband was having elective hand surgery --I dashed across the street to make use of this waiting time efficiently. Mammograms were once again annual for me after two lumpectomies for ductal carcinoma in situ (DCIS) in 1990. After those two surgeries I was advised that no special follow up was needed other than mammograms every six months for the first two years. Those years had passed uneventfully, and I had returned to annual mammograms. I also stayed on my hormone replacement therapy (HRT) as the doctors assured me that there was no link between DCIS and HRT.

The eleven years had flown by. My husband and I enjoyed our rural coastal community in northern California where we walked by the crashing Pacific Ocean waves. Our dream house was built close enough to the bluff top that we could fall asleep at night to the sound of the waves breaking on the rocky shore beneath. Our children were all raised and busily pursuing their respective careers. Grandchildren were born and, although not living close enough to be "hands on" grandparents, we loved visiting them nonetheless. Travel had become a big part of our lives and we were particularly fond of cruising -- with trips getting longer and longer. In fact, the elective surgery my husband was having that September day was carefully planned between the trip from which we had just returned and the one coming up later that fall.

Dressed in the usual paper gown ("Take everything off from the waist up and put on the gown. It opens in the front") I waited in the hallway while the mammogram was read by the radiologist. Because I had time to spare before my husband would be released from the hospital surgical unit, I had invited a friend from high school to meet me at the radiology office so we could grab coffee after my "routine" visit. I found myself absently turning the pages of a very old Sunset magazine paying no attention at all to the articles when the radiology technician returned. "We need to take some more pictures." As she led me back into the mammography room she explained. "The right breast (where I'd had the previous surgery) showed something." "They want to get a better picture." This had happened once before when they had obtained a new machine, that had produced an abnormal picture (called an artifact). I was still unconcerned. I gladly shed my gown once more and submitted to the squeezing of my breast by the jaws of the machine. As the tech squeezed tighter, she asked, "Are you ok?"

"I am. Tighten down even more if you need to. Get a good shot." She was quick and efficient and I was soon back in the hallway waiting area with that slow old Sunset magazine.

When she returned, I was so primed to hear the tech say "Everything's' ok" that I could barely comprehend it when, instead, she said, " We need to do a ultrasound and see what this is. It wasn't there a year ago." I was led into a small dimly lit room and put on an examining table. Mary, the technician then put on gloves; spread the ultrasound gel over my breast and with the machine humming began to scan my right breast. She moved the "wand" over my breast in circular motions and would stop and click the computer keys when she wanted a picture taken. I assumed after a couple of "clicks" that I would be done. But, she scanned and scanned. For the first time I began to wonder if something was wrong. Was she just unsure of herself, I thought, or was she finding so much that she had to take many pictures? After what seemed an eternity, she announced, "Sit up while I go over these with the radiologist". By now I was concerned that my friend in the waiting room was done waiting.

When the door opened, Mary had returned with Dr. Poojoolian, the radiologist. He introduced himself, shook my hand and announced, "We'd like to take you over to the other side of the building and do another ultrasound on a machine with higher resolution. We see the original source of our concern, which is definitely just a cyst, but Mary has found another, smaller mass, which we need to examine further." With no time to respond, I was off the table and headed out the door.

"Oh, wait, I said, My friend is in the waiting room and I want her to come with me." I think I expected a negative answer, but instead Mary opened the door, called out to my friend, and off we went to "the other side."

My friend Helen is a physical therapist. When we started college together we both wanted to go into nursing. Helen eventually chose physical therapy and I stayed with nursing. We had remained friends,

3

but not close throughout the subsequent forty-three years. Yet, instantly we bonded again when I told her what was happening. She, like me, is not afraid to ask questions of the medical profession and at times we were both questioning what was happening. Another technician appeared in this new ultrasound room and we were crowded. Dr. Poojoolian told Mike, the technician, "Start scanning at 11:30 on the right breast." He started at the 11:30 position. I could see a nickel size round circle on the monitor. Dr. Poojoolian turned the monitor and explained to Helen and me, "This is clearly a cyst. I am certain because it is translucent and very symmetrical."

"Mike, scan toward an 8 o'clock position (very much closer to the nipple)." As Mike scanned, Dr. Poojoolian ordered, "Stop - there it is." As Mary, Mike and Dr. Poojoolian all looked and said "hmmm," I could feel my pulse begin to race. Helen spoke up and asked, "What does hmmm mean?" They turned the monitor, and the doctor explained "Here we have a smaller, dark, asymmetrical mass." " You have a couple of options. Both options involve the next step, which is to determine whether or not the mass is benign or malignant. You could return and I will do a needle core biopsy where a needle is inserted under local anesthesia and several "punches" made to get specimens of the mass, or you could go back to your family doctor and be referred to a surgeon who might just take the tumor out." I opted for the former for two reasons: I was impressed with Dr. Poojoolian and his explanation of what he was visualizing on the ultrasound. I also figured that by staying with Dr. Poojoolian , I could get the procedure done sooner than by going back to my family practitioner and starting from scratch.

When we returned to the original side of the building and, after dressing, Mary said, "I'm very glad that I took so long in doing the ultrasound."

"What were you doing?" I asked.

"I scan the entire breast when asked to do an ultrasound rather than just scanning the area where the original shadow is located. I'm often told that I take too much time doing this --that I should speed up. But, today it really paid off."

"I want the earliest appointment I can get." They worked me in at 1:00PM the following Wednesday.

Helen and I left the radiology building and made our way across the street to the hospital to find my husband just coming out of anesthesia. His first words were, "How was the mammogram?"

I replied that "I'll tell you on the way home."

He said, "There's something wrong, isn't there?"

Knowing he was groggy with anesthesia, I replied, "I'll tell you as we drive home; we have two hours to talk."

He dozed off and Helen and I had a chance to chat and she agreed to go with me to the needle biopsy the following week. As Gordon's eyes fluttered open again, he repeated the same question, "How did the mammogram go - is there something wrong?" When I tried my same answer, he pushed harder, "I have the feeling that something is wrong." Again, I promised details as soon as I got him safely in the car and on our way home.

Good to my word, I explained what had occurred during the time that Gordon had been blissfully asleep under anesthesia. My explanations were punctuated by Gordon's periodic sleep from the effects of his surgery. But, surprisingly, he would awaken every 20 or so minutes with full retention of what I had said. We both agreed "the sooner the better" for the needle biopsy.

Do I call my five children or not? That was my next question. I wanted to forget it until I knew something, but that's not me. I problem solve best by talking through situations and this was certainly no different. One son is a lobbyist for the California Medical Association and his wife is a nurse. They are the most knowledgeable members of the family on health matters so I started with them. But, at this point, we all agreed. Don't panic and start thinking malignant when you don't know. So, although I told most of the family, I said that we would just enjoy the weekend and await the Wednesday appointment.

Wednesday was a beautiful fall day and the drive down the coast was lovely. No hint of trouble in the air. As Gordon went off to a hand therapy appointment, Helen and I lingered over lunch at an outdoor table, basking in the fall colors. At precisely 1 0'clock, we were in the waiting room. I fully expected that they would let Helen come in as before, but I was disappointed when they informed me that the procedure would be done in the very small original ultrasound room that could barely hold three people and the equipment. Helen promised to wait for me until Gordon returned. What a super friend!

The needle core biopsy was performed much like the ultrasound only using sterile technique. Mary did the tasks that didn't require a sterile technique and Dr. Poojoolian was gloved and proceeded to wash the skin of my breast with antiseptic, use a local anesthesia on the skin and then slowly insert the needle. He used one hand with the needle, and the other hand to guide the wand of the ultrasound over my breast to locate the mass. He turned the monitor so he could see, but I had to have my head in a position that made it impossible for me to see. There was no discomfort at all. However, when Dr. Poojoolian located the area where he wanted to get a specimen, he said, "Ok, you will hear the trigger on the needle." BAMMMMMM - the noise was frightening and I jumped. For such a quiet procedure, the needle "punches" sounded like he blew the breast right off my chest.

"Can I see the specimens?" Puzzled by this request, Dr. Poojoolian let me sit up to see six pinkish gray pieces of tissue about a centimeter long. "Interesting but they Don't look very threatening" was all I could say.

"We'll have an answer by 1PM tomorrow."

The specimen was sent "across the street" to the hospital pathology laboratory. They would call Dr. Poojoolian who in turn promised to call me. Mary gave me the "inside" phone number where I could call if I had not heard by 1:30PM.

CHAPTER II
BACK TO THE PAST

So far, so good. I could handle 24 hours. While we wait for the diagnosis, let me tell you my background. You have some time, right? This might help you understand my reaction to the rest of this story. As I mentioned previously, I am a nurse. I went to nursing school at Stanford University after two years at the University of California where I received an AA degree in physiology. Never excited about the hospital environment, I found my passion in public health nursing. My first job after graduation was with the Santa Clara County Health department where I had a caseload that consisted of many migrant farm labor families. I loved making home visits into the rural areas of the county and learned as much from these hard working families as I taught them about preventive health. I eventually moved to the state's capitol, Sacramento. After receiving my masters degree in Public Health Nursing Administration, my career took a twist as I started teaching instead of administering. I became first an Assistant and then an Associate Professor of Nursing at California State University, Sacramento. I loved helping students find a zeal and passion for helping people help themselves - not in the sickly hospital environment, but in their own homes. I loved teaching. And then, yet another career twist occurred. Since my nursing department was so close to the state capitol it was only natural that when issues regarding baccalaureate nursing arose, we went to the legislature to lend our expertise. I was never interested in politics, and was therefore astonished to be "selected" to travel to the capitol for the purpose of lobbying a state legislator who was authoring a bill that we did not like. What I found during those first and subsequent visits was that lobbying was much like teaching, and hence very much like my previous preventive public health work. I found legislators generally open to being "educated" on an issue about which they had no particular knowledge. After several months of such trips to the capitol from the classroom, the state nurses association asked if I would take a full time position with them as a lobbyist. As this was 1976, women were very much in the minority among lobbyists. And nurses basically considered politics beneath their dignity -- and I include myself here.. And yet, I had witnessed first hand the possibilities for educating the people who controlled my profession through the bills that were passed and signed into law. But, I hated leaving the security of a tenured faculty position that I dearly loved. After much thought I struck a compromise. I would take a "leave of absence" from the university for one year --with the option to extend it to two years-- and lobby. After that period of time, surely I could decide where I wanted to be.

Lobbying was a tough business. Thrilling, exhilarating, frustrating and upsetting - -and that was only the first day. I quickly found that in the health care field, medicine was king with a capitol K. Nursing had, previously, only a part time male lobbyist who was better at wining and dining than teaching about nursing. Such had been the "usual" method of lobbying. A legislator gets a lunch, and/or dinner, a game of golf, another dinner and then a friendship is established. Within these "friendships" the business of lobbying took place. Nursing had a very small budget for lobbying, let alone wining and dining. I had no idea how to crack this male dominated profession. By attending and testifying at committee hearings, I was soon known at the capitol as "the nurse." But, the very first legislator whom I had been sent to lobby from the university saw my brains and my vulnerability. I took him to lunch as my first ever attempt at the business of wining and dining. When the bill arrived at the end of the meal, he offered to pay.

"Oh, no,. I'll pay." I wanted to be the sophisticated lobbyist and I proudly signed the bill and wrote the nurses association name on it.

The waiter came back and said that "I'm, sorry, madam, but you are not on the authorized account list." I wanted to fade into the cotton pillows of the booth that we shared. The legislator came to my rescue and paid. Back at the office, the problem of authorization was quickly put to rest; no one's fault, just naivete.

But it was not just wining and dining that was difficult. I was up against other lobbyists when it came to testifying before committee hearings and I had to be aggressive enough, verbal enough and able to think on my feet. Slowly, I gained the respect of other health- field lobbyists and the legislators. So much so that at the end of the first year, I opted for the second year's leave of absence. At the end of the second year I had decided to become a legislative candidate myself.

Political affiliation was never an issue as a lobbyist, so when the seat representing the district where I resided became available, I took that first legislator out to lunch once again. By now, sophisticated and sure of myself, I asked him what he would think about me running for office. He was surprised and admitted he had no idea about my political party. After we established that we belonged to the same party, he offered to introduce me to the "operatives" who assisted candidates.

It was the spring of 1978 and I was 39 years old, mother of five, nurse, and associate professor of nursing -- planning to throw in a run for office. The problem was, once again, my naivete. The fifth assembly district was a heavily Democratic district and I was a Republican. No Republican had won for many years there and no woman had ever succeeded. By the time the filing was over, 12 Democrats were running plus 2 Republicans- me and a college student even less polished than I. I thought that the Republican Party would finance my run, as I was proud to stand up and run for such a difficult seat. It was delicately explained to me that: 1) money was not put into races that could not be won and 2) I had never been one of the Republican Party regulars - in fact all I had ever done was vote. I was unknown - -a nobody.

Pride and determination would not let me back out. I had friends help with homemade signs and pamphlets. Primary election day saw the Democrats beating each other up, while I sailed to victory in the Republican primary. The run up to the general election in November was a different story. Shortly after the primary, one of the party operatives asked "What is your base?"

I said, "Pardon me, I don't know what you mean." He explained that a base was where my money and support would begin and who would that be? Again, I had assumed it would be the party. He just laughed. But I was mad. I explained that there were 180,000 registered nurses in the state and I guessed that they were my base. His reply? "Get $1.00 from every one of them and you'll have yourself a race." I took him literally and began to appear at every nursing function that time would allow. Fellow nurses held coffees and fundraisers. My legislator friend helped open doors for me too. Slowly the money came in - not at $1.00 per nurse, but more like $20per Registered Nurse. The "operatives" were impressed. I walked precincts with my kids and found it fun. Later, I was to discover that legislators hate to walk precincts. But I didn't know that. For me it was similar to the home visits that I had made as a public heath nurse; only this time, I handed them a pamphlet insisted of collecting a urine sample.

Well, Election Day was amazing. In a 64% Democratic district, "the Republican nurse" won with 62% of the vote! I became the first nurse elected to the California State Legislature.

Once elected, I had a constituency of 350,000 people-- just like a large caseload. These were my people with needs and concerns that needed to be addressed. I opened a district office that had the caring and feel of one of my former health- care offices. In my capitol office I was now lobbied and I worked there four days per week. My committee assignments included Health Committee and there I heard many people testify on many proposals during my eight-year tenure. I also chaired the committee on Aging and Long Term Care, where I was privileged to carry much of the early legislation relating to Alzheimer's disease. But, the greatest impact that I made on public policy during 1981-82 came from my constituent Candy Lightner. A repeat offender drunk driver killed one of her twin daughters and from this horrible accident the organization MADD (Mothers against Drunk Driving) was born. I worked with Candy and introduced legislation that determined how the state would deal with drunk driving in general (blood alcoholic levels) and how to deal with repeat offenders. The progress in California stimulated like-minded people in other states and this awareness changed the perception and penalties for driving drunk. This for me was the high point of my career. It proved that one single person could make a difference. The Candy Lightner story was a made for TV movie that is still running today. I learned that no one should feel powerless to bring about change.

After my fourth term in office I chose not to run again. I had just married Gordon (the kind and thoughtful legislator that I met on my first trip to the Capitol). I wanted to devote time to the marriage and to my family. For a few years after that, Gordon and I formed a government relations firm. However, much of my time was spent as a keynote speaker. I spoke to many, many groups about how to get involved in government and how to bring about change.

CHAPTER III
BACK TO THE PRESENT

By 1988 we decided to move to the rural north coast and become active in volunteer activities. It was there that I was first diagnosed with ductal carcinoma in situ.

I returned to Sacramento for my annual mammogram expecting to get the results in the mail. I was somewhat surprised when my gynecologist called and told me that she had just received a report stating that I had "micro-calcifications." She explained. " These are very small particles that appear on film as though someone has poured a shaker of salt into the right breast."

Although I did self-breast exams on a rather haphazard basis, these micro-calcifications were too small to be detected by touch. She referred me to an oncology surgeon in that city.

Dr. Ramjet wanted to do a maestecomy immediately for two reasons. One, he believed that breasts were nothing more than fat and therefore unnecessary. Also, second, that he "could sleep better at night knowing that any chance of cancer was destroyed." I was so angered by Dr. Ramjet's offhand attitude towards my body that I sought a second opinion. A thin volume that I had read came to mind: "Keeping Abreast." It was put out by a study group through a major health center in San Francisco. I found that I could obtain a second opinion there. A pathologist would review all my mammograms and offer advice as to the minimal treatment of choice. From this visit, I o concluded that I needed only a lumpectomy. Dr. Ramjet had a good reputation as a surgeon and was amenable to doing only a lumpectomy, so I decided to stay with him. But, he could be very intimidating and rather condescending. I felt empowered by the second opinion, and told him what kind of treatment I wanted. Actually, it took two surgeries, because I insisted that the first be done under local anesthesia. Frankly, I didn't trust the doctor to perform just a lumpectomy and not a total mastectomy. Dr. Ramjet did not get all the micro-calcifications out on the first surgery and I returned for a second lumpectomy one month later. At that time there was no further follow- up, other than mammograms, as most cancer specialists considered micro-calcifications in the ducts as pre-cancerous. I then transferred all my health care files to the city closest to our coastal location and considered that chapter of my life closed.

One of the bonuses of retirement was being able to embark on activities that I had long delayed. I was intrigued with a Jane Fonda tape that focused on weight lifting for woman. As Jane is only a few months older than I am, she became my role model for beginning weight- lifters. Gordon was amazed when I asked for a weight bench and free weights for my birthday and even more surprised when I actually began a regular lifting regimen. I combined this twice a week activity with step aerobics from a Kathy Smith video.. But, perhaps my greatest challenge occurred when a friend told me that a group of senior women were starting a tap dance class. The local dance instructor had agreed to take on a group of nine women from ages 53 to 70 who either had never danced, or had not tapped since childhood.

I was the youngest, but had no tap dancing experience. We were terrified of the teacher and so for the first year, she assigned us to a less intimidating instructor. Only later did we discover that the intimidation worked both ways. The beautiful and very talented studio owner, age 40, had no idea how to relate to these older, questionably talented, but very determined women. Our grit and determination paid off as we traveled thirty miles each way to class twice a week for ten years. We became "The Gingers" and performed up and down the California coast. We became pioneers for other middle to older age coastal women, and several other classes began based on the wonderful fun and camaraderie that we exuded. Our "piece de resistance" was in San Francisco at Finoccio's nightclub. There we danced as back up "chorus girls" for a gorgeous drag queen. Our signature costumes, different for every performance, consisted of fishnet stockings and fringe on our leotards. We savored appearing a little risqué, when we actually had on more layers of clothing than usual. Public appearances like this were a far cry from my previous civic life where speeches were delivered in sincere suits of black, gray or proper navy blue! With my body more on display, I turned to more serious weight lifting. At first I had a personal trainer who instructed Gordon and me once a week. Soon we bought gym equipment and established a room in our house as the gym. It seemed natural to begin instructing others who were interested in weight-lifting and soon I had eight regular students whom I taught in the home gym. Later on, the community was fortunate enough to get a certified aerobics instructor and of course I had to try that out as well. Ten years after my original lumpectomies, I was in better physical, mental and emotional shape than at any time in my life.

CHAPTER IV
TODAY

Have you waited long enough to discover my current diagnosis? Is it a return of the microcalcifications? We fast-forward to the present (September 2001) and the 24 hours of waiting is almost up. I called Dr. Poojoolian's office and was told that the results were not in, but due any moment. I sat by the telephone -- sort of praying, sort of trying to assess how I would take either verdict. The phone rang and Dr. Poojoolian started with,

"I am very sorry to have to tell you..........it is invasive ductal carcinoma." He indicated that surgery would be the next step. I asked him whom he would recommend, knowing that he would defer to my family doctor to help me decide. I asked if I should go to the University of California, San Francisco and again he agreed that I should do whatever I wished. This was not extremely helpful, but I understood that it was my decision. I then asked if I had time to take a trip that we had planned for October. He was more specific on that one: "if you must go, then go, but it would be better to postpone your trip and have surgery."

I hung up feeling confused and disoriented. I knew no surgeons in Santa Rosa, the nearest city. I didn't know if I started by talking to an oncologist, or a surgeon. I called my number three son, a police officer, who had told me that his chief's wife had just gone through breast cancer surgery. As they live in San Rafael, closer to San

Francisco, I surmised that they would have some information regarding doctors there. He promised to get right back to me.

Meanwhile, I had a meeting of a women's circle to which I belong. We number ten, all between 50 and 65 years old and all searching for deeper meaning in life. We have been meeting for 2 1/2 years every two weeks and have become quite close. The closeness is of the mind and spirit in our common quest, although we do not necessarily see each other socially. I arrived a little late, which is frowned upon as we each take five minutes to share with one another our joys, sorrows, and concerns from the previous weeks. When they asked me to take my turn, I started to cry. I didn't know that I would cry -- I'm not the crying type, especially outside the confines of my own home. They hugged me and let me talk. I was interrupted by my cell phone (another no,no, but forgiven this time). It was Glenn with a list of references from the police chief and his wife. Within the space of two hours, this son of mine had a reading list for me plus the names of doctors and hospitals. After calling my number two son, the lobbyist for the California Medical Association, I was in good shape to make some choices, or so I thought.

I went online to the University of California and saw that I would need a referral to get an appointment into their cancer second opinion clinic. And of course, I researched many web sites about invasive cancer.

By Monday morning I had the " bible" of breast cancer, Dr. Susan Love's <u>Breast Book </u>and a fair idea of how I wanted to proceed. I made the call to my family physician. I could get right in to see him and off I went. Immediately he told me that my health care plan, an HMO(Health Maintenance Organization), would NOT allow me to go out of the area for a surgeon, oncologist or even a second opinion. He gave me the name of a surgeon, a woman, that he felt was very good and the name of a male oncologist. I still couldn't understand who came first, the surgeon or the oncologist. "I'll send in the referrals to your HMO and then you can make appointments after they are approved." " I'll want a second opinion," I said. He flat out told me that a second opinion would not be approved, but that I could try. Our small clinic does have a person who gets the referrals made, and so the visits were planned to the surgeon and oncologist. The referral person called and argued with me that it was pointless to ask for a second opinion until I had a first opinion. I argued back that with the time lag involved, I "would have the first opinions before getting the second." She reluctantly agreed to send in the request to my HMO. Meanwhile, my options were to pay privately or to wait. No physician or University was going to see me before the payment mechanism was clear. I asked myself about the fortunes of someone in my situation who didn't have the option to pay privately.

As the weeks began to pass, I was reading everything that I could find about breast cancer. And as I gathered information, I thought back to my original diagnosis in 1988. I wondered if my records were available, and if so, if I could obtain them. By sheer luck, my former surgeon's office had them stored in archives and faxed them to me. By law, they only needed to have been saved for seven years, so I was fortunate to get them. I saw that the pathologist, Dr. Michael Logan, had been my "second opinion pathologist" at that time. He was the one to encourage a lumpectomy instead of the mastectomy that Dr.. Ramjet wanted to do as a cure for his own insomnia.

I had no idea how to find Dr.. Logan at this time, but on a chance, I typed his name into an Internet search engine Bingo! Dr. Logan was still in San Francisco and had narrowed his practice to just doing second opinion breast consultations. I couldn't dial the number fast enough. Yes, I could private pay for his second opinion. He would get all the slides from the hospital, and then we would set up a conference call after he had faxed me his findings.

After the approval for the oncology visit arrived, I was told by that doctor's office that I would have to wait about six weeks to be seen. I begged to be called if a cancellation occurred -- and, it did. My husband and I traveled the two hours for that visit full of hope, expectation and armed with all my medical records plus my new found cancer knowledge.

CHAPTER V

MEETING THE ONCOLOGIST AND THE SURGEON

During the visit, I found Dr Dick to be very thorough. He told me that he would write down on yellow ledger paper what he was telling me and that way I could read and re-read everything at home. He laid out all the possibilities:

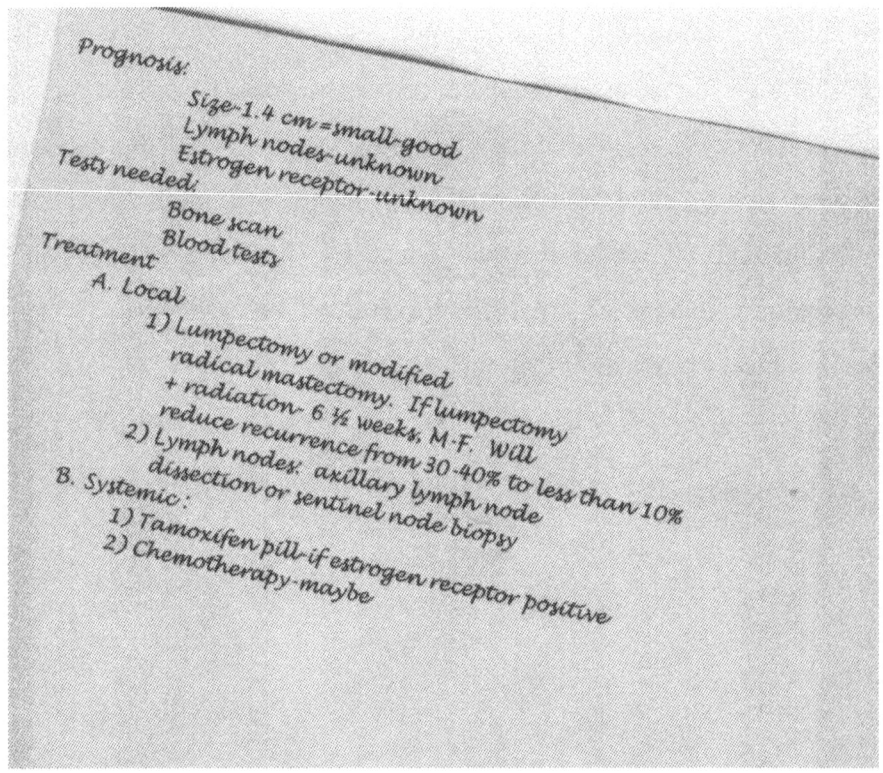

Prognosis:
Size-1.4 cm = small-good
Lymph nodes-unknown
Estrogen receptor-unknown
Tests needed:
Bone scan
Blood tests
Treatment
A. Local
1) Lumpectomy or modified radical mastectomy. If lumpectomy + radiation- 6 ½ weeks, M-F. Will reduce recurrence from 30-40% to less than 10%
2) Lymph nodes: axillary lymph node dissection or sentinel node biopsy
B. Systemic:
1) Tamoxifen pill-if estrogen receptor positive
2) Chemotherapy-maybe

I appreciated this thorough discussion of all the possibilities, although I was quite certain what I wanted, based on the research I had done, if the blood tests and bone scan were negative. Dr. Dick explained that those tests were being done to see if the cancer from the ductal carcinoma eleven years ago had spread into my system or whether this was a new occurrence. I then asked him about my greatest fear --not breast cancer, but Alzheimer's disease. I told how I had watched my mother's ten-year decline due to that condition. I had been witness to and a participant in moving my mother from home to facility to facility as her condition and finances worsened. I do not wish to travel that path as a patient and certainly do not want to have my children feel as helpless as I did.

"Studies are showing a strong correlation between estrogen intake and the prevention of Alzheimer's and conversely, the increase in those women who did not take hormone replacement therapy (HRT)" I said.

But, Dr. Dick suggested, "Not enough research has been done, and I cannot condone the taking of estrogen if the tumor is estrogen positive." I decided not to push that point.

Between the time of my oncology visit and my first visit to the surgeon, I received the first report from Dr. Logan. We had a one-hour phone conversation after he sent me his review of my needle biopsy slides, plus reviewing all the past history of 1990.

Dr. Logan 's report said, in part, "In the absence of a prior history of radiation therapy for the ductal carcinoma in situ, this patient has the therapeutic option of an adequate excision and sentinel node procedure followed by radiation therapy. Given the grade of the carcinoma, and not withstanding the 14mm size noted by ultrasound examination, there is only a small likelihood of nodal involvement and I believe a sentinel node procedure would be adequate."

It's a good thing that my nursing school vocabulary came back to me so that I could understand most of what that report actually meant for me. Basically, Dr. Logan was telling me that since I had not used up my once in a life -time chance for radiation, that I could have it now. That was the "therapeutic option" or opportunity for treatment that he was suggesting. The use of the words, "nodal involvement" I recalled referred to the lymph node system. Most of us know that we have lymph nodes under the arms and in the groin. Actually the lymph system is a complex system which I will study up on further. But I needed to know now is what Dr Logan meant by "sentinel node biopsy."

Sentinel node biopsy is a pretty straightforward procedure whereby a blue dye is injected into the breast at the site of the cancer tumor. This dye then moves through the nearby lymphatic system to the closest lymph node to the cancer site. This is the lymph node that is also most likely to have drained any cancer cells spreading them through the system. That first draining node is called the sentinel node and it is removed and studied. Since the sentinel node is closest to the tumor, it is a good predictor as to whether or not the cancer cells have spread to other nodes. If the sentinel node is normal, there is a low chance that a positive node will have been overlooked. However, not all surgeons are trained to do this procedure and many want to remove the nodes that extend deep under the armpit. (Perhaps this also has to do with the surgeon's need for sleep at night?)

I raised the question of estrogen and Alzheimer's disease with Dr. Logan. "I think that taking estrogen after surgery is quite appropriate, because of several new studies that show that breast cancer survivors are no more likely to get recurrences with HRT than those with no HRT."

He cited a new study out by Dr. Ellen O'Mara, from the University of Washington. "Dr. Dick wants me to go off estrogen."

"Why don't you go see a doctor who specializes in menopause."

"There is someone who specializes in menopause?" I retorted.

"Dr. Kay in San Francisco. Talk the whole hormone question over with him."

So, I now had at least established that I wanted a lumpectomy with sentinel node dissection. If the surgeon and I were compatible, maybe I wouldn't be so adamant about a second opinion. And I felt that Dr.. Logan was my best second opinion from a pathology standpoint anyway.

Three days later I met Dr. Sweet. From the minute that her staff allowed Gordon into the room with me, I figured that we were off to a good start. Dr. Sweet came into the room with great speed and carrying all my mammograms. She shook hands with both of us and said, "Let's see what these mammograms show." When I told her that the mammograms wouldn't show anything, she looked at them through the x-ray view box and then said, well, let's look at the ultrasound.

Up went the ultrasound and she said, " Ok, here it is. I recommend a lumpectomy and axillary node dissection. I have one opening for surgery in two weeks."

I immediately agreed to the date, but explained that I wanted sentinel node dissection instead of the entire axillary node dissection. I explained that I had talked with Dr. Logan.

"I know Dr. Logan and, I respect his opinion. But I am not comfortable removing only the sentinel node. I want at least one other node out also." As this seemed a compromise between total axillary dissection and the sentinel node only, I accepted it. Two nodes: one sentinel and one axillary. I liked Dr. Sweet. She was open, friendly and said she respected my desire to keep as much breast as possible. She also agreed that the most difficult part of many breast surgeries is not the breast, but the arm and shoulder aftermath of nodes being removed. Thank goodness for the *Breast Book* by Dr. Susan Love, for it had been my first resource with regard to axillary nodes. I had followed that resource with another book, *Uplift* by Barbara Delinsky, that contained testimonials by different woman. I had learned that the taking of nodes is like taking away part of the body's sewage plant. The lymph system is a huge recycling network. It collects "garbage" from the body and strains and recycles at lymph node sites located throughout the body. Once this recycling is complete, the fluid is returned via the bloodstream to be used again. What an efficient system! The lymph nodes also recognize anything that is foreign or threatening to the body in this process. When this occurs, the lymph nodes hold onto this material in order to develop antibodies to fight off whatever is occurring. Therefore, in breast cancer it is important to identify which lymph node in this complex system is draining cancer cells. Confirming that nodes are negative means that the cancer has not spread. But, since nodes do not regenerate, the removal of many nodes compromises the lymphatic system forever.

I had recently attended a high school class reunion where a classmate showed me the difference in the size of her arms. Pulling up the sleeve of her jacket, she revealed a left arm that appeared to belong to a woman twice her size. Amy explained to me that this was called lymphedema. She experienced the swelling a few weeks after her breast cancer surgery. The pain was horrible at first, far worse than anything experienced with her cancer operation. Her doctor had told her that "to make sure there was no spread," (and as you now know, so that he can sleep at night), he had performed a full axillary dissection. He said that she was lucky that all the nodes were negative. But now, five years later, she still covers her arms in long sleeves and takes other precautions. She cannot carry her purse over her left shoulder. Her blood pressure can't be taken on the left arm, and long plane trips are out. All of these activities compromise the few lymph nodes remaining on that side and cause tremendous swelling and then pain. This problem is so common that there are even lymphedema organizations, not to mention the many web sites devoted to this chronic condition.

I wanted to be able to return to aerobics and weight lifting without any arm or shoulder stretching or mobility problems. I was determined to have only two nodes removed.

CHAPTER VI
SURGERY

Guess What? My second opinion request had been denied by my HMO stating that I did not need to go to San Francisco for another opinion, as there were specialists present in the community where my oncologist and surgeon were located. This was no great surprise. I gave up that fight, partly from fatigue and discouragement, and partly because I had received Dr. Logan's counsel, which I considered a second opinion.

The surgery was set for the local hospital. Two days before, the admitting nurse called and took my history. When we went to check into the hospital the morning of my surgery, I checked the admitting form. It said, "partial mastectomy with axillary node bisection." I said, "Oh, no!!" I explained that I was having a "lumpectomy with sentinel node dissection." A call was made to the surgeon's office and the form was changed. My nursing and legislative days had taught me well - don't sign anything that is not what you mean. But this was disturbing. I thought that once the doctor and I had an understanding of the procedure, that it would be communicated to the office staff. Apparently, it had not been passed along and if I had been too nervous or scared that morning to read the surgical consent form accurately, I could have had the wrong procedure.

The preoperative period was easy. Many patients were being prepared for surgery at the same time and so, with only curtains separating one from another, you could hear why everyone else was in the hospital. No one else used the word, cancer. My pre-op nurses were great. They talked with me, kept me warm with blankets from the microwave, and allowed my husband to stay with me. I was only concerned that I had not met the anesthesiologist and surgery was due to start in 30 minutes. With only fifteen minutes to go, I was wheeled to another section of the hospital. There, in another large room, were about 6 patients, all with paper hats, paper slippers and stripped of anything that could fall out, such as teeth, glasses, jewelry. My husband was still with me when the anesthesiologist finally came in. He reviewed my history. I told him that I was prone to "overreact" to drugs and did not want to feel "hung over." He said that with the new drugs, that would not happen. Within minutes, a male nurse took me into the operating room. The scrub nurse was counting the scalpels and other sterile equipment, but turned and greeted me as I scooted from gurney onto the operating table. The surgeon came in and that was the last I knew.

Awakening in the recovery room was just like waking up after a good night's sleep. I felt awake and fine. My breast was bandaged and I had a drain attached from tubing coming out of the bandage. The recovery nurse asked questions and I responded as though we were all friends. She warned me not to let the pain "get ahead of me" and suggested I accept some pain medication. I felt no pain, but agreed. The phrase, "Don't let the pain get ahead of you" was used over and over again. And yet, no one had really explained how much pain was the point where I should worry. Dr. Sweet briefly stopped by. "I'm going to talk to your husband. But everything looks okay." She would have the final pathology results the next day prior to my leaving the hospital.

After the great care received in the post -op setting, it was a shock to be moved onto the regular nursing ward. I was taken to a two-bed room, where fortunately, the other patient was out. I was offered lunch- - and as I was starving, I happily agreed.

My hospital stay was fine until ten o'clock that night. I had felt so good that I had been up, put on makeup to greet my family and two friends who came by. I had been accepting the pain medication every four hours and had no pain. But, just as I thought that I would settle down to sleep, the worst happened. A very elderly lady, awaiting surgery was moved into my room. Her previous roommate was suicidal. This lady had been in the hospital several days for tests. She was crabby and demanding. They told her that they had to start blood and that the machine would be brought in shortly. So, my anticipation of sleep was gone; bright lights were turned on, voices were loud and got louder while talking to this hard of hearing, cranky woman. I began thrashing around trying to sleep and slowly began feeling worse and worse. Thinking that this must be from lack of sleep, I asked for more pain medication as I thought that would relax me and put me to sleep. Instead, every time I closed my eyes I saw bright, swirling lights and felt dizzy. Getting up to the bathroom, I found that I was very nauseated. By then it was almost seven in the morning and the cranky roommate was yelling for the nurses - she refused to use her call button. I finally asked for some crackers, as I knew that otherwise I would be sick. When breakfast came I could barely look at it let alone eat it. My husband and daughter arrived ready to have me discharged. I felt AWFUL. I told the nurse I was very nauseated and she said, "Oh, we have something for that - we'll put it into your IV." The only problem was that it caused uncontrollable sleepiness as it took away the nausea. I fought the sleepiness, as I desperately wanted to see Dr.. Sweet and get discharged. But I knew that the 2-hour ride home was going to be miserable unless I felt better. I struggled and struggled to stay awake.

Dr. Sweet appeared and she was distraught. A very close friend had died suddenly the night before and she could hardly keep herself together. She told me that she would remove my drain and discharge me and then she too was going home. "The report came back, negative nodes -- no spread of the cancer to the lymph nodes. The tumor was estrogen receptor positive and I got it all out." With that, she was out the door and I was glad to let my eyelids close for a bit.

Getting dressed and getting discharged were only difficult because I just wanted to sleep. My daughter drove me home so that my husband could detour and grocery shop. Once home I slept for three hours. When I awakened I felt fine and refreshed. The lesson I learned was that only I could judge my pain level and when asked, "Where is your pain on a scale from 1-10?" I didn't know how to calculate. To be on the safe side, I had taken the pain medication and that coupled with little food and no sleep made me sick. Even now it is difficult to calculate for pain is such an individual experience. Some scales suggest the nurse should ask from 1-5 with the higher number representing intense pain. The 1-10 scale, called the Visual Analogue Scale starts at 0 indicating no pain and increases to 10 being the worst possible pain. The difficulty is not with 1 or 10 but figuring just exactly where you are between those numbers.

My recuperation was uneventful and eight days later I had back-to-back appointments with the oncologist and the surgeon. I approached the appointments full of optimism. Little did I know that I was soon to have the worst day of my life.

CHAPTER VII

CHEMOTHERAPY, TAMOXIFEN AND OTHER POST-OP DECISIONS

Dr. Dick pulled out the yellow tablet as soon as we were seated in the examining room. He said, repeating from the first visit, that he would write this all out so that I could have it upon returning home. He started with my diagnosis and proceeded to outline the size, the lymph node status, and the estrogen receptor as positive.

"There is extensive ductal carcinoma in situ and the margins are close but negative. Clean margins are necessary to insure that all the cancer has been removed."

I had no idea what close but negative really meant.

"Your prognosis is 85% cured. Now I'll write out your treatment."

"I want to ask about the ductal carcinoma and the margins."

"Please not interrupt me until I am done". I felt as though I had been slapped in the face. He then proceeded with his treatment plan.

"Systemic treatment needs to consist of immediately stopping hormone replacement therapy (HRT)." He underlined the word **definitely.**

"You'll go on Tamoxifen (a drug that hopefully prevents breast cancer) twice a day for five years. Side effects are hot flashes (15%) and uterine cancer (1%) and blood clots (1%). Taking the Tamoxifen and stopping the HRT would improve my prognosis from 85 percent to 90-92 percent.". I attempted again to interrupt and bring up the

O'Mara study that showed that cancer survivors who continued on HRT did no worse than those who stopped.

He snapped, "That was not a randomized study. Please do not interrupt me."

Now I was getting mad. I couldn't ask questions, I couldn't talk and he was increasingly speaking to my husband and not to me. He then offered me chemotherapy if I wanted a 2 percent greater survival- - i.e. to 92 percent. Of course, the side effects would be hair loss, fatigue, and low blood count among other things. I replied with great certainty. "For 2 percent I could get hit by a truck."

But the real shocker was yet to come. Methodically putting all this down on the yellow lined paper, Dr. Dick said, "Now we will discuss *local treatment.*

"You need further surgery to get better margins due to the extensive DCIS (ductal carcinoma in situ) and that could be another lumpectomy or a mastectomy."

I was floored. All my ability to discuss my future rationally went out the window.

"More surgery?" I asked.

"Yes," he replied, " and followed by 6 1/2 weeks of radiation."

I was numb, but I went on to my next question and asked about doing a hormone level test.

"Couldn't we find out what my hormone levels are now, and then with those results, add enough estrogen or progesterone or whatever I needed to get rid of the menopausal symptoms?"

I had been getting less and less sleep at night and I was pretty sure that it was due to lack of estrogen. Dr. Dick said that Tamoxifen would act like a mild estrogen to all the body except the breast and that should help. He asked me, "What would a blood test show except that you are post menopausal?" Another slap in my face.

I left the office with tears running down my face. My husband, who had so rarely seen me this upset, didn't notice at first and asked, "Where shall we go for lunch?" Only when I snapped back at him did he realize the extent of my dismay. I thought that I was going to the doctor to hear that with my tumor out, the nodes negative and radiation coming up that I was fine and could go back to living normally. More surgery? I just couldn't believe it. Thank goodness I was seeing the surgeon immediately after lunch.

Arriving at the surgeon's office, I got the comeuppance of my life. After refusing chemotherapy without hesitation and making that comment, "For 2 percent increase in survival rate, I could be hit by a truck," that is *"exactly what"* happened. As I pulled into the parking spot in front of the doctor's office, a truck hit our car. Not bad, but enough to involve the usual insurance hassle and a rental car for several weeks. I couldn't believe it. I felt as though God had turned his back on me.

The surgeon, Dr. Sweet, said, "I don't think that more surgery is needed, but will defer to the radiation oncologist to see if she needs cleaner margins for radiation."

By cleaner, the medical profession means more space without any disease. There is a minimum area needed for radiation to be most successful. I hadn't even been referred to a radiation oncologist at this point, but agreed to get this other opinion. Once again, I was dismayed that this health care system with which I felt so familiar seemed so woefully disjointed. Dr. Sweet faxed a hand written note to the radiation oncologist and asked her advice. They would get back to me.

As we were planning to go to Scotland for that country's spectacular New Year's celebration called Hogmanay, I knew that I could not have another surgery plus radiation before the end of the year. I had read, and even Dr. Dick had confirmed that radiation could be delayed as long as six months. I decided that we were going to Hogmanay - no matter what!

The next day, the radiation oncologist called.

"I sent the surgeon's fax on to the pathology department at the hospital. They had a different pathologist than the one who did the original slides take a second look. His opinion was to do further surgery, just to be sure." Foolishly, I did not get a copy of that report.

Within fifteen minutes, the surgeon called me and said that she had a noon surgical opening later that week.

"Do you want to take it or risk the chance that I won't have another opening through the end of the year?" This rush for surgery before the end of the year was due to another drama that was being played out by the doctors and the insurance companies in our county. I was a member of an HMO (Health Maintenance Organization). Therefore, the use of this doctor was dependent upon whether she was a part of the providers in that HMO group. A great number of the specialists in that HMO had refused to sign a new contract, and were going to be off contract the end of the year. So, I grabbed the surgical opening and planned for another surgery, ever mindful of the December insurance deadline when my doctor would no longer be available to me.

Meanwhile, in checking with my local family doctor, I discovered that patients were in a panic about their coverage. It was true -- this particular HMO was losing doctors. My husband and I began looking at our insurance options. We found that we could change immediately to a PPO (Preferred Provider Organization) that would allow us far greater medical choice, at of course, far greater increase in cost. Worried that we were up on the deadline to change health plans, we jumped to a PPO as of the first of the year. The insurance fight continued. It was editorialized in our local paper. My surgeon wrote a scathing letter to the editor, and we, the patients, felt caught in the middle. For me, I literally *was in the middle,* between surgeries, between health plans, and between treatments. Great! One's plenty.

When I pulled myself together and took many deep breaths, I put in a call to Dr. Logan. I figured that I would get his opinion on whether this second surgery was really needed. His office got back to me , telling me that he was out of the country on a speaking engagement, but that he had taken a quick look at my request and suggested that I wait seven days until he returned. But, the seven days fell AFTER the scheduled surgery date.

Again, worried about the December insurance deadline, I decided to proceed with the second surgery -- with one caveat. I refused to stay overnight in the hospital, opting instead to stay in a local motel with my husband as my "nurse." I figured that at least I wouldn't have a cranky old roommate who was having a blood transfusion. I also reasoned that we were only a short distance from the hospital if an emergency arose. My husband was a little nervous, but supportive of my decision.

The second surgical routine was a re-run of the first. By now the pre-operative nurses knew me and were friendlier. I had the same terrific nurse in post-op. Once again, I came out of the anesthesia clear-headed and when Dr. Sweet came by, I asked, "What did you find?"

"Nothing -- absolutely nothing." I thought that she meant there was no more cancer, so I wasn't concerned. Within a few hours, and without any pain pills other than Excedrin, I left the hospital for the motel. I had the drain in place and an appointment the next day to have that removed before we headed up the coast for home. Gordon was a great nurse. He pampered me and let me eat whatever sounded good. I slept much better in the motel than in the hospital, and was anxious to have the drain removed. The visit to the doctor's office was eventful only when she removed the bandages and I looked. She commented, "This incision leaves you more disfigured than the first."

"I didn't realize what you would look like sitting up as you obviously are on your back during surgery." The incision line now goes right through the areola and pulls the entire nipple up and over towards my armpit. Good thing my topless days are over. As the days turn into months, however, this disfigurement bothers me more and more.

CHAPER VIII
RADIATION

Now that I was home with no further surgeries to contemplate, I needed to see the radiation oncologist to get that part of my treatment scheduled. I had to decide whether to have conventional radiation, which would take up to seven weeks, or to try the newer brachytherapy radiation, that would be concluded in just one week. I got an initial consultation appointment within two weeks with a radiation oncologist who used conventional radiation only. So, I needed to do my own research again to be sure about the option that was best for me.

Brachytherapy is a type of radiation that is fairly new to the treatment of breast cancer. I discovered it through a chance statement from the pathologist, Dr. Logan. When I mentioned that I would have to leave my home for almost seven weeks to have conventional radiation treatments in a neighboring city, he said, "Check out brachytherapy." I asked him to spell the word, as I had not heard it before even though I thought that I was rather current on breast cancer treatment. I have to say that the fastest and most up-to-date method of checking on treatments or drug options is to do research using a computer search engine. When I did so, a wealth of information opened to me on brachytherapy.

The treatment as been used for many years with prostate cancer. Brachytherapy is now being utilized in other parts of the body.

Basically, this is a method of delivering radiation to the body by the use of implanted seeds in the case of prostate cancer, and by the use of plastic catheters in breast cancer. I learned that the closest center to my home that was using this treatment was a medical center one hundred miles away. The reason I read further was that radiation by means of brachytherapy was completed in five to seven days. That's right – seven days instead of seven weeks. I couldn't read fast enough. I quickly calculated that I could possibly accomplish brachytherapy before my end of the year trip to Scotland.

Many web sites explained the procedure in basically the same way. Plastic catheters about the length of crochet needles would be implanted around the tumor site (under anesthesia). Ideally this would be done at the time of the original cancer surgery. However, sites noted that since not many centers were doing breast brachytherapy, most patients required a new surgical procedure to insert the rods. After insertion of these rods, they remained in the breast for the entire week of treatment. The radiation is administered via a linear accelerator into the catheters once or twice per day for a few minutes each session. After each session, usually completed in fifteen minutes, the patient was to spend the day in rest and relaxation. Because of the protruding catheters, a patient could not wear tight clothing and therefore was restricted to wearing lose and flowing garments. Some of my reading suggested that most patients spend the week either at a site on the hospital center grounds dedicated to out-patients, or alternatively, in a hotel near the center. I definitely got the idea that you didn't feel like too much movement.

The idea of reducing seven weeks into seven days prompted me to call the medical center in Northern California where breast brachytherapy was being provided. I received prompt and thorough information about how the procedure was done at that center. A packet of information came to me along with an extensive questionnaire. I made two initial requests:

1) I wanted to speak to a radiology surgeon who actually performed the catheter insertions;

2) I wanted the names and telephone numbers of at least two patients who had gone through the procedure.

I was very impressed when the doctor called me almost immediately. He explained the procedure, stating that I would have to have another operation to insert the catheters. I would then rest for one full day before the radiation would begin. I was beginning to get excited about this and so called both Dr. Dick and Dr. Sweet to ask their opinions. Dr. Dick: " I don' know much about it, but it can't hurt to check it out. Dr. Sweet: " I really know very little about it. Why don't your call Dr. Tomlin the radiation oncologist who would be in charge of your conventional radiation?."

Dr. Tomlin was much slower to return my call, but when she did she spoke against the breast brachytherapy on the basis that it was too new and untried in breast cancer cases. That of course only made me more interested.

I received the names of two patients who had completed breast brachytherapy. One was a forty-seven-year-old professional who undertook this method for the sake of expediency. She lives in the city where the procedure took place. The second patient was a sixty-seven-year-old woman who was retired and just felt that she would become less fatigued if the radiation were competed within a week's time. Both women had excellent reasons.

The first patient described her week as "a week from hell." "I had to drive to the medical center with the catheters protruding from my shirt. I couldn't sit straight as the bottom rods would jab into my chest wall and the pain was acute. The only position that was half-way comfortable was to be semi-reclined. And I had to maintain that twenty-four hours a day!" Sleeping was almost out of the question as she reclined in a big chair. Walking was restricted due to the catheters bumping her chest, her arm and anything else in sight. It would have been ideal to have someone else drive to the medical center, but her husband couldn't be available every day. When I explained that I would be coming to the big city to stay in a hotel for a week, she began to laugh. " Well," she said, "bring plenty of valium and lots of videos that you want to watch, because you won't be good for anything else."

I asked her again about the pain.

"It was considerable. I took pain medication for the entire week. After the last day, another minor procedure was performed to remove the rods. Six months later, I still had some scars that were not thoroughly healed."

I realized that I had not considered the condition of the skin that would be somewhat compromised by the radiation catheters.

However, this patient did agree that seven days from "hell" got her treatment over and done with in a short period of time.

The second patient was able to describe a less traumatic time. Her retired husband took her to treatment every day. She too had to "sleep" in a chair but didn't seem to mind and found the pain only "minimal." There was something in the tone of voice of both women that began to put me off on brachytherapy.

The insurance coverage was going to be another interesting component of breast brachytherapy. Because I was still under a Health Maintenance Organization (HMO), I could guess at what their answer would be. And I was correct. They would not pay for me to go out of my area to receive a "different" type of radiation when the accepted treatment was available to me in the nearest large city. I had already signed up with my retirement plan to change my health insurance at the end of the year to a Preferred Provider Option (PPO). This was going to give me less coverage (80%) than the HMO (100%) but would allow me to obtain care in whatever medical center I chose. So, at this juncture, my choice to obtain brachytherapy would be out of pocket or wait to have the procedure done when my health insurance coverage had changed at the New Year.

My decision was fairly simple. If I could not complete my radiation before my trip in December, then the reduced treatment time of brachytherapy lost its appeal. Having come to that conclusion then, the seven weeks of pain free traditional, well-documented radiation, sanctioned by my physicians, won out over the more maverick breast brachytherapy. My insurance would pay 100% of the cost and I was able to have the tattooing, that I will describe later, performed before I left on my trip.

I encourage others to research new options for treatment as they become available. The Internet is a wonderful resource, if only to get some primary information. No one is going to put the right health care treatment plan together for you better than you can do it for yourself. Remember, doctors did not go to medical school to become teachers. Doctors want to treat not teach. You must take care of yourself and be comfortable with your decision. The thought of a week in a nice hotel watching videos still has great appeal, but I made the right decision for me. Sometimes, though, my decisions didn't jibe with traditional treatments.

For instance, I decided that I did not want to take Tamoxifen as I could see no guaranteed benefit and lots of potential problems for perhaps a 5 percent increase in survival rate. I decided that I would try "natural soy" products in an attempt to get just enough estrogen to stave off the potential for Alzheimer's disease, which continues to be my bigger fear.

I had frankly always laughed at the friends who felt afraid of estrogen and who drank and ate "weird" things in order to get "natural" soy. I found myself biting my tongue as I called a couple of them and asked for their advice. I tried powdered soy (ugh!) chocolate flavored powdered soy (a little better), and liquid soymilk (umm good). I tried menopausal vitamins, high doses of Vitamin E, kava, kava and melatonin, St. John's Wort and something called "Herbal nightcap" that included dried passion flower, alfalfa leaf, hops flowers, dandelion leaf and chamomile flowers. And then I started hearing stories about how soy, due to its estrogen content, was suspect in the area of breast cancer too.

I was again concentrating on hormones and no longer thinking about cancer when I had my first appointment with Dr. Tomlin the radiation oncologist. She had studied my history thoroughly because she mentioned my several careers as we sat down in her office. During her initial questioning about my diet, she asked, "Do you smoke?

"No."

"Have you ever smoked?"

"No." I was patting myself on the back at this point

But then, next question, "Do you drink?" I told her that I enjoyed a cocktail every night and occasionally a glass of wine.

"You should give that all up. There is a strong correlation between alcohol and breast cancer. Well, a couple of glasses of red wine, per week, for your heart, maybe.

I thought, "Oh, no, here we go again!" The rest of my diet measured up, but my supplements were questionable. She explained that once I started radiation that I should stop Vitamins A, C, E, and selenium, as I need "oxygenation" and should not be taking anti-oxidants.

"What about Tamoxifen?"

"I don't want to take it and I want to take estrogen". She frowned and warned me that was a very dangerous idea. I let it pass. Dr. Tomlin then explained "On your first appointment you'll would have "tattoos" and "simulation." Plan to be here for 2 1/2 hours. How soon can you begin?" When I said that I was going to Scotland for Hogmanay, she asked "Couldn't you postpone the trip?" My husband started to answer, when I quickly said, "No, New Years cannot be postponed. We are going." With a shrug, my answer was accepted. Leaving this appointment, I got a booklet on radiation. "We'll call when a simulation appointment becomes available." Reading the radiation booklet with the mention of a side effect of cumulative fatigue convinced me that postponing this treatment until after our trip was very wise.

The oncology office called several days later informing me that they had one appointment available - 2:00 pm *"on my birthday."* We had not planned to travel to "the city" that day, but figured that we would go out for a nice birthday dinner and spend the night in the city at a luxury hotel (the proverbial make lemonade out of lemons). The procedure went just as described.

"Take off everything from the waist up. Put on a gown. It opens in the front. Take a seat in the patient's waiting room." I was placed on a large gurney type bed and told that the tattoos would be tiny and permanent. They are placed so that each time I would have radiation, the technician would know exactly where to place the beam. The tatoos would be the outer limits. If a washable substance was used, I could get radiated in different locations if the markers wore off. The technician that afternoon was a woman who seemed cold and indifferent. I couldn't believe that she didn't notice my birth date as she went over my chart. Looking rather forlorn, I suspect, my picture was taken with a Polaroid camera. I was to see that ugly, sad picture every time that my chart was opened from then on. I never asked why they needed my picture dressed in the hospital gown, but I later heard the following reason.

At the University of California Medical Center in San Francisco, a very wealthy socialite was scheduled to have radiation. She was told that she would have this "mock up" session where measurements would be taken and she would be positioned for her up coming treatments. She decided that she did not have time for such a simulated session, and so sent her maid in her place. When the technician called the woman to undress and don a gown and get in position for the simulation she noted that the "patient" was of a different race than the woman named in the chart. When the technician asked the woman, "Are you Mrs. X?" the woman hastily answered, "No, I am her maid." The technician of course rushed to tell the doctor who called the patient on the telephone to explain that substituting one person for another did not work. The linear accelerator is programmed very specifically for the measurements of the individual patient. And so to insure that this scenario never was repeated, the Polaroid picture of the patient was initiated. The picture is then affixed to the chart, which is present during each and every radiation session.

Then I was placed in several different positions, all on my back with my arm over my head. My arm was out of the sleeve of the gown enabling me to reach as far back as needed. The room was cool, and I was instructed to keep my head still and stare straight up to the ceiling. If I needed to talk, I was to talk to the ceiling and not move my head. The technician left periodically and several others wandered through the room. No one offered to cover me up when they left and no one inquired as to weather I was cold or not. Dr. Tomlin came in twice to "check the measurements." This "simulation" is just like having measurements taken for a form-fitting shirt. Everything must fit just perfectly. The same was true for the tattoos for these would be the outside marker giving permanent testimony that I had received radiation. Because radiation can only be given in one area of the body once during a lifetime (usually), these markers must be permanent. Finally, I was through, I thought. But, no, I was told to take my clothes out of the locker and proceed across the public corridor to another public waiting room for the CAT scan. As I grabbed up my clothes, I hoped my bra wouldn't drop out from under the shirt into the middle of the busy hallway. Sitting in a waiting room where everyone else is clothed and you have only a gown tied around your waist is embarrassing. I was juggling clothes, my purse, a bottle of water and a magazine - all the while trying to look casual and confident. "You mean you don't have this done everyday?" At last a male technician called my name and ushered me into yet another changing room where he told me to set my clothes. He then picked up the chart and said, "HEY. Happy Birthday."

What a difference that made. We began to chat.

"What are you going to do to celebrate?" And then he told the female tech who entered. I felt suddenly happier, warmer and ready to cooperate. They positioned me for the CAT scan, and it went without problems.

"Thanks for noticing that it's my birthday. But don't figure out which birthday!" Such a little kindness, but it meant so much. Arranged my appointment for the first radiation treatment: January 28, 2002. I was told that it would be at 10:30 each day. Monday through Friday for 30 treatments followed by 3 "boosts" that would bring the total number to 33. I was not offered a choice of time, just told the procedure.

Now I only had two lingering concerns. What had Dr. Logan found after reviewing the pathology slides from my second surgery? Was on-going hormone therapy going to happen? I was now taking up to nine ibuprofen at night to get to sleep and to stay asleep. I set up an appointment with Dr. Logan for another telephone consultation and made an appointment with my family practitioner to discuss hormones.

Dr. Logan started the conversation with "Why didn't you just wait seven days until I returned? You didn't need the second surgery!" He went on to say that the two millimeter margins were sufficient and that the review of the pathology slides showed no DCIS in the tissue removed during the second surgery! I had made a big mistake. Caught up in the panic of health insurance changes, end of the year surgery schedules, and my own tendency to want things over and done with, I had rushed into a needless surgery. No particular harm done except a very disfigured breast with a nipple that looked like it was trying to hide under my armpit. Matched to the other breast that was drooping with age, I was going to need Victoria Secret and the magic air filled bra to look halfway normal.

I then asked Dr. Logan, "What about the admonition against drinking?"

He replied, "Do you have a liver problem?"

" No, no" I was quick to tell him, but Dr.Tomlin had said a high correlation existed between those who drink alcohol and breast cancer due to the fact that alcohol stimulates estrogen.

Dr. Logan is always great with the relative risk factors.

He explained that the largest study is by a researcher named Francheschi from Italy. In women age 50 to65, over a fifteen-year period, the expectation is that 5 out of every 100 women will get breast cancer. With moderate alcohol consumption there is a relative risk of 1.4 percent. Multiply that out and you have 7 women or an additional 2 in a 15-year period. Dr. Logan concluded "You have already been one of those women. On the other hand, there is a 10 times greater risk of dying of vascular disease and from Alzheimer's." He suggested that I continue to enjoy my single malt scotch and not stress about it.

"Okay, I can do that."

CHAPTER IX
HORMONES

Next, I decided to get serious about the hormone question. I picked up a new book called *The Wisdom of Menopause* by Christine Northrup, MD. In it she reports that blood testing for hormone levels is not very accurate, but that saliva testing is quite accurate. In the appendix, she lists several laboratories that do such testing. One laboratory was within one hundred miles, so I gave them a call. They promised to send me all the information that I needed on different hormones that can be checked by one test. I was told that in my state, California, I would need to have a physician order the tests. Perfect. I had an appointment to see the doctor in a couple of days. I read all the information and decided to have the following hormone levels checked: estradiol, estrone, estriol (all estrogens), progesterone, testosterone, DHEA, cortisol and melatonin. The three estrogens and the progesterone results would tell me exactly how much of these I am producing as a postmenopausal woman. As pre-menopausal woman produce testosterone, and I had previously been taking estratest, that is, an estrogen with testosterone in it, I was just curious about that result. My reading had informed me that DHEA and cortisol work in opposition to one another. Cortisol is the "fight or flight" hormone and too much of it is a positive indication of stress. Chronically elevated cortisol levels represent ongoing stress over an extended period of time and are detrimental to health. Extended high levels have been associated with excessive bone breakdown. Checking my melatonin level would tell me whether or not my sleep deprivation was related to low melatonin or to low estrogen levels. As sleep deprivation was my most disturbing symptom, I was anxious for these results. The laboratory informed me that all but melatonin was collected upon awakening in the morning. The melatonin specimen had to be collected at 2:00 am, as it is time specific. The 2:00am didn't bother me, as I was so frequently awake at that time anyway. The laboratory employee took my Visa card, as my HMO does not cover this service. They then sent out the vials and instructions. My family practitioner was interested in what I was trying to discern, and I promised to bring in the results as soon as they arrived. About two weeks after collecting and mailing the saliva specimens to the lab, my results arrived. They consisted of graphs that showed normal levels for each of the hormones, and then my level. The results were surprising. My estrogen and progesterone levels were low, as one would expect, but my testosterone level was off the chart high. My cortisol level was elevated indicting the stress and surgery that I'd been through and so its counterpart, the DHEA was a little low. The melatonin came back perfectly normal. My interpretation of all the data indicated that I need some estrogen. I carried these results to my family practice doctor. He surprised me with his reluctance, and then outright refusal to prescribe estrogen.

"How about giving me only the estrogen vaginal cream? That would be a very modest dose." He refused.

"You need to deal with another issue--that uterine bleeding that occurred with the low, continuous dose of progesterone that you had previously been taking. Maybe you should see the menopausal specialist in San Francisco." I was very, very disappointed. I wanted to try the vaginal estrogen and then retest to see if my levels and symptoms were better.

Christmas was coming and with it the entire family and grandkids would be gathering at our home. It was a busy, hectic wonderful time, but made difficult by the sleep deprivation. I was grumpy and cried for no reason. As we were leaving for Scotland on Dec 27th there was no time to see Dr. Kay, the menopausal doctor in San Francisco. I called and scheduled an appointment for January 28th, three days after I returned and the first day of my radiation. I forwarded all my medical records to Dr. Kay.

Then on December 21st, the most wonderful surprise occurred. My family nurse practitioner called and asked how I was doing. I told her that I was doing terribly due to sleep deprivation caused by the low estrogen level.

"Why don't I order a low dose vaginal estrogen?" This sleep deprived zombie burst into tears of thankfulness.

With the prescription filled, my husband and I left for Scotland. I began to sleep and sleep and sleep. No more flashes, lots more sleep. It was like a miracle.

CHAPTER X
RADIATION TREATMENT

When January 23rd, 2002 rolled around, I had almost forgotten about breast cancer, surgery, drugs and radiation. I felt good. But, I knew I had to finish this journey with 33 days of radiation.

Way back last fall I had heard that the local hospital, in conjunction with the County Assistance League, had several apartments and homes that were rented out for an incredibly low amount to people who lived out of town. As we qualified as "out of town" due to our 4-hour drive, I had put my name on the list. We were told not to count on it, as when an apartment was given to an out-of-towner, there was no push to limit their time. So, we had made plans to house sit at a friend's house for a couple of weeks, then stay in a motel the remainder of the time. I had researched short-term rentals but there was nothing. It was a complete surprise then to find a message on our answering machine, after an absence of a month, that an apartment was available. At $15/day, we were somewhat wary of what it would be like, especially since when I asked what I should bring along, I was told, "Your toothbrush. Everything else is there."

Everything else was there: a fully furnished 2-bedroom apartment, complete! Other than adding fresh food to the refrigerator, nothing else was needed. We quickly unpacked our clothes and I headed for my first radiation appointment. Gordon and I were both seated in the "front" waiting room and after a short wait, a tall, gray haired man in a lab coat called my name. He ushered me back through a narrow hallway that is flanked with a window looking out unto a central garden area. A quick turn to the left and I was in front of a set of lockers and little cubicles or "cubbies." He explained that I should take a cotton gown from the clean stack, and use one of two changing rooms. "Take everything off from the waist up. The gown ties in the front." Then I was to put my clothes in a locker, lock it, put the chain around my wrist and take a seat in the Patient's Only waiting room. I did so.

As the room became a focal point for me during the next 6 ½ weeks, I'll describe it in some detail for you. The patient's waiting room consisted of eight chairs, four on each side of the room facing each other. At the end opposite the entrance, there was a built in shelf where coffee, water and cups were placed. There was a magazine rack with current issues of *Time, Better Homes and Gardens, People* magazine and several others. Beside one set of chairs there was a low end table with a bowl of hard candies. At the other end of those chairs was another low end table that filled the space between the chair and a small, rectangular shaped window that viewed the garden. The entrance was open and directly off the hallway where I had entered from the front office. The middle of the room was empty. I entered and took a seat. There were two men already there; one fully clothed and one whose gown barely covered naked knees and legs. This man was older and obviously uncomfortable, as he kept trying to keep his gown closed. The younger man looked up and said, "Good morning, how are you today?" I answered the proverbially, "Fine," but found myself uncomfortable at talking to someone so fully clothed. A very efficient looking woman dressed all in white and carrying a clip board entered and spoke directly and only to the clothed man explaining to him that his father would take longer that day, due to the fact that he was having x-rays taken along with his radiation. The clothed man then turned and in Spanish, told HIS father what had been said. "A-ha." So now I understood why the clothed man was in the patient's waiting room. I felt better, although treated by the lady in white as though I was invisible. At that point the man in the lab coat returned, and said, "We're ready for you, Jean." He led me just beyond the changing rooms and through an open room where several computers and TV monitors sat at standing height long tables. I was led hard left into a large room with the linear accelerator in the middle. Lab coat introduced himself as "Dakota" and said that he would be the technician working with me today. I was told to take my right arm out of my sleeve and to lie down on the gurney that is attached to the linear accelerator.

He explained, "Your pillow is made of plastic and your right arm will be in a plastic armrest above my head." Dakota inserted a kneepad under my knees once I was lying down and in place. My view was of two red lights in the ceiling. "Again when you talk, keep your head in place and talk to the ceiling. If you have to move or sneeze and the technicians are out of the room, wiggle your fingers and the machine can be stopped." Dakota then proceeded to take out a green felt marking pen and begin to mark me. Additional marks that would wipe off, but were applied every day in order to line me up with the previously prepared numbers on the computer screen behind my head. Dakota casually told me, "Well be doing this each day," and he put marks on the nipple, on the breast, on my chest. The pen felt cold and bothersome. I asked, "What do you use the permanent tattoos for?"

"Those are the outline parameters," he explained. "These today are where the dose is actually aimed." I still didn't know why I needed the original and permanent tattoos if I was going to be "lined up and marked" every day. My breast was pushed down, my gown was pulled under me, and a small ruler was placed on my chest right beneath my breast, all in this lining up process. Well, I thought, if it takes more time today, surely each day will go faster as they have all these numbers figured out. Finally the accelerator itself started to move into position. With a humming sound, the two large spheres, on opposite sides of me began to move into position. Dakota explained, "The first position will be for 40 seconds and the beam will be coming from the upper left side and into the breast from that angle. After that is finished, I'll come back to the room and rotate the accelerator so that the second beam of 80 seconds will be coming from the lower right side. The beam is basically under my armpit."

He continued, "In a couple of weeks, you'll have no hair under your arm pit, only a sunburn."

Terrific, just what I always wanted. Finally, the positioning was done. Oh, I almost forgot - as he did the measuring and marking, the lights were off in the room so that he could see the lineup visualized by a red beam that came from the machine. Once he was ready to

leave the room and turn on the accelerator, he turned the lights on. The room was actually nicer with the lights off, but I was not going to ask too many questions this first day. Dakota left the room. I wondered if I would know when the process started. I stared and stared at the two red lights over my head. My knees felt tense, my whole body felt tense. I told myself to relax - imagine the ocean - imagine just floating on a wave. My reverie was interrupted by a loud BUZZZZZZING - as though a huge swarm of bees had been unleashed. I'm sure I jumped as I realized, "Oh, this is the radiation - this is it." After what seemed a short time, there was silence - and then the big metal door opened and Dakota appeared. "Don't move," he said, "but we're half way done." He directed the movement of the spheres to my other side by using hand held controls. I had no further markings, but the sphere was fitted with a plastic device with slits in it and a piece of cement in the middle with wing nuts that Dakota tightened. He then took something that looked like a plug and inserted it into the sphere.

"OK, here we go," he said, walking out the door. A few seconds later, I heard the hard thud of the door closing. This time I was prepared for the buzzing sound, but found that 80 seconds was a long time just staring, so I began to pray. I prayed that God would help me through this time and promised that everyday I would use my radiation seconds to try to listen for God's words to me. This prayer time became, for me, much bigger and more important than the radiation that was going on around and into me.

Dakota burst into the room and said, "OK, put your arm down, and you can sit up as soon as I get the table lowered." Grateful that my abdominal muscles were still strong enough to allow me to pull straight up into a sitting position, I was up and off the table. I got my arm back into my sleeve and was leaving the room when another technician, a woman, told me that now we would set up my appointments for the next 32 sessions. I looked surprised and told her that I was informed that 10:30 was my time and that it would work well for me. She then explained that every new patient gets the 10:30 spot for the first day, but then are assigned their regular time. "Why was this not explained to me earlier?" Of course, she didn't know. She told me that for the remainder of the first week, she would have to move my appointments around, but that from the start of week two, I could have 10:15. Good, that would work. As if I really had any choice. I was given one appointment for 3:30 that week plus two 5'oclocks. I was very glad that I was not driving back to the coast every day or that I didn't have a work schedule, or children to be picked up. I was then informed that I should go back into the Patient's waiting room and wait for "the nurse" to talk to me about skin care. When I explained that I had another appointment in San Francisco (1+ hours away), the tech responded that I could see the nurse another day, but to remind them as they might forget. I was walked to a cubbie which now said "Jean D" on a new piece of labeling tape. "Keep your gown in there from Monday to Friday. After your Friday session, place it into the "used gown" hamper and pick up a clean one on Monday." I was also told that some people want to keep the same

gown and, take it home to launder themselves. I can't imagine that I will become that attached!

CHAPTER XI
A MENOPAUSAL SPECIALIST

At 11:15, we left for San Francisco. An unusual cold front had moved through the area and snow was on the ground right down to the freeway level. It was truly amazing and beautiful, as we very rarely have snow, let alone on the freeway. The storm had passed and the ride was uneventful. We were anxious to see Dr. Kay, menopausal specialist.

Visiting medical offices in San Francisco is quite different than in small rural cities where we are accustomed to parking close to the front door at no charge. The first task in a large city is planning enough time to find a parking garage that has an opening. Fortunately, the large garage near the medical center had a vacant spot. Navigating the medical building was the next order of business and we had to laugh, as we couldn't locate the office; the restrooms, yes, but the office no. We were thrown off by the fact that the number was a 100 number indicting the first floor, but there were a pharmacy, a minimart and a couple of other shops there also. When we found the correct office number, it was the closest office to the street; in other words, so easy to find that we overlooked it. We were early and the door was locked so we split a sandwich and sat outside with a mix of building employees and other patients doing the same thing. At exactly 1:00pm, the door opened, revealing a very small but sophisticated office. The colors were mauve and cream with flowers in a large black vase. The woman who opened the usual sliding glass counter window gave me a questionnaire to complete. Nothing too unusual about that, until I looked at the questions. Instead of the usual, "What are your previous surgeries? What did your parents die of?" the questions were related to diet, sleep and feelings of well-being. There were perhaps fifty such questions. I could tell immediately that this physician knew what my problems were all about. I filled in my history of disrupted sleep, fuzzy thinking, and moodiness. I also watched the patients that were arriving. All women, all late forties, all dressed very "city sophisticated." I anticipated a long wait, but shortly was called in. I asked that Gordon join me and that was totally acceptable. We were put in "the study" - a very small room with a desk, bookshelves and not much else. Within seconds, Dr. Kay appeared. He was physically short, elderly, with a beard, glasses and an earring in his left ear. He was dressed in shirt, tie and slacks. My first impression was that he looked not like a physician, but more like a jeweler. Neither white coat, nor stethoscope draped around his neck. He joked about which one of us was the patient, and then sat down at his desk. I was seated looking straight at him, while Gordon was sitting behind him. He opened my chart and I could see the cover letter that I had sent to him was underlined in several places with two colors of ink. He passed by my letter, moved right to the current questionnaire and said, "You need to add more fish to your diet." "The alpha omega oils are very necessary for good health; you live on the coast, so fish should be easy to obtain." We then had a short talk about fish being difficult for us to get as all that was commercially caught went to larger markets than where we reside. But, I promised to increase fish into our diet. Then he looked me straight in the eye and said, "Mrs. Duffy, what do you want?"

My instant reply was, "I want to feel like I did a year ago; energetic, emotionally stable, able to sleep through the night."

He said, "You can have all of that. Just go back on your estrogen." He went on to say that there are nineteen studies, involving 1,512 people with up to a 38 year follow up, which show that HRT (hormone replacement therapy) after breast cancer does not adversely effect recurrence and/or survival compared with controls. He pulled a reprint off his bookshelf, underlined it and handed it to me.

"Your symptoms are all consistent with estrogen deprivation, " he continued, "and there is no scientific reason for you not to return to HRT." I explained what all my doctors had said, including the fact that Dr. Dick, the oncologist, had said that the O'Mara study was not a randomized study. "Of course not," he said, "We can't subject cancer patients in the United States to randomized studies. That would mean taking a group of post breast cancer women and giving some of them estrogen and similar numbers a placebo. You cannot do that to people in this country. Patients, who either have or have had cancer, have a right to choose and to know what they are taking. Therefore, all the studies are comparative and anecdotal. But, the numbers are consistent." He pulled another study off the bookshelf and pointed out the findings to Gordon.

"My family doctor worried about more uterine fibroids if I should just take estrogen."

"No, no, he explained, "you take progesterone for two weeks every eight weeks and when you stop, you will bleed. The reasoning is that by bleeding, the uterine lining eliminates the buildup from estrogen and therefore the potential for uterine cancer. Since this is an artificial cycle, the length of time between cycles can be determined by how much bleeding occurs. If very little, then the progesterone can be used every 12 weeks or so, if the bleeding were heavy, the progesterone would be taken more often, perhaps every 6 weeks." He concluded by saying that he would send a letter to my family physician stating this regimen should be tried. He suggested that if breakthrough bleeding occurred, as had been my problem last year, that a sonohystergram be scheduled. When I asked what that was, he referred to a sonohystergram as a "water ultrasound." I would need to research that one.

At 2:00pm we were back in the car and I felt as though I had my life back. I couldn't wait to get back to my estrogen pills. The feeling of euphoria was wonderful. I felt strong and empowered. I felt like maybe now I could stop "fighting" the system and get back to normal. As my pills were home, 150 miles away, I would have to wait until the weekend to get started, but I was happy at just the thought.

CHAPTER XII

THE RADIATION EXPERIENCE A WEEKLY JOURNAL

Radiation, day number 2 was at 3:30 in the afternoon. After complying with the routine of changing into my gown, putting clothes into the locker and entering the waiting room alone, I found another scene. Seated across from me, fully clothed was a very efficient looking, petite woman of about 35 years old. When a large young woman dressed in the uniform of an employee (white pants, blue smock) came in to refill the coffeepot and change the water, she started a friendly conversation with the other woman.

"How are you today, Anna?"

"Oh, my husband is getting 2,500 calories through the feeding tube. My nursing background is really helping us." They chatted like old friends. I was completely ignored. Then, a young, nice looking man with a gown covering a naked chest came from the radiation room. I could see that his neck was very red and his jaw appeared swollen. As the women chatted about how he wasn't losing weight, he interjected through clenched teeth and with obvious discomfort, "Yes, but when you can't taste any food, and the food bypasses your stomach, you are constantly hungry."

"Oh, but you get sips of water," his wife reminded him. I think how lucky I am.

I tried to keep that good feeling with me, as I am called for my radiation not by Dakota, but another man. This technician is named

Gavin. He is East Indian and was born and raised in Fiji. His accent was very difficult to understand. I didn't get all of his background on day number2, of course but I'd like you to understand my sense of betrayal (almost) at finding yet another man to mark my breasts with the ink pens. He was very quiet and mannerly. I asked, "Where's Dakota?"

"Dakota works four ten hour shifts as he lives in another city, whereas I live locally so I work five eight hour shifts." As the door slammed and I was alone, I vowed to use the time in prayer. I decided to recite The Lord's Prayer and see if I could do it in 40 seconds. When Gavin reappeared to shift the machine for the second position, I asked him about the cement wedges that he secured with the wing nut. He explained that those are barricades preventing the rays from getting where they are not to be. The plastic shield to which it is attached has slits in it, which direct the rays through the breast. Once again I was amazed how low-tech that seemed in comparison to the rays themselves. When the door slammed for the second time and the 80-second treatment began, I decided to try and recite the 23rd Psalm, which I had not said since my childhood Sunday school days. I realized part way through that I had forgotten much of it and would need to bring a Bible from home and refresh my memory. Soon, the treatment was over.

On Day number 3, I was told to arrive at 5:00pm but if I would get there at 4:30, I could see the nurse about skin care. Wanting to understand what I could do to prevent burning, we arrived on time. Sitting in the outer waiting room we watched the clock approach

5:00pm. The nurse, Natalie, finally showed us into a room. She was the lady whom I had seen previously who looked very professional and efficient always clad in white pants, shoes, shirt and sweater. She carried a clipboard and pen and looked ready for anything. She assured me that we would get through what she had to say before my 5 o'clock time, but nevertheless left the room to take care of another matter. Frustrated and annoyed we sat and watched the hands of the clock. With about five minutes to spare, Natalie returned and started a routine that sounded as though she was very bored, ready to go home, and that her mind was elsewhere.

"Stop taking antioxidants. Your skin will get more and more red and could break open into oozing sores. However, radiation can't be stopped, so use aloe vera or this. She handed me a sample and discount coupon.

"Don't wear underwire bras, because anything touching the skin will get increasingly irritated. Stop shaving under that arm." As I stood up and stated that I'd better go, she turned on the friendly charm, as if she realized that, her routine speech over, she saw us as real people. We were pleasant, but left the room and this time I told Gordon to come to the patient's waiting room, as everyone else seemed to have a partner there with them. As I entered the waiting room minutes later in my gown, there was a fully clothed woman in a wheel chair and a man seated behind her. The woman had her head down as though reading the book that sat in her lap. She was probably in her 40's with long dark hair that partially hid her face. She appeared to be tall and very thin. The man also appeared to be reading, but he was turning the pages quite quickly in a nervous sort of way. No eye contact was made with us and I was reluctant to start a conversation. Suddenly there was a great pounding of footsteps as a woman approached down the hallway looking very agitated. She looked in at us and then proceeded right towards the monitors where the technicians were standing. She was stopped there, "What are you was doing?" "Where is my sister," she demanded. I heard a tech ask the name of her sister and then she was told, "She'll be out soon." The woman, dressed all in black, threw herself into a chair with a loud, exasperated sound. Seconds later, she jumped up and began pacing back and forth in front of the window to the garden. Meanwhile, perky Natalie the Nurse, clipboard in hand descended on the woman in the wheelchair, saying,

"Now, you must tell Dr. Tomlin about your depression. You must get some sleep." I looked up dismayed that this personal problem was being discussed in front of three of us. Why couldn't Natalie talk with the woman in the privacy of the examining room? Gavin called me. My turn for radiation.

Day number 4- my appointment was again at 5:00pm. When we arrived (and I now had Gordon come back to the patient's waiting room with me), I see that the "depressed" woman in the wheelchair was there; as was the "sister" still attired all in black. I no sooner had changed than another woman came from the changing room and the "sisters" leave. The woman in the wheelchair continued to read, her eyes never looking up as various people walked past. The husband remained seated behind her and also appeared to read. As good as I am at finding an opening for conversation, none existed with these two people. I wondered what she had. But, I'm called again by Gavin and off to radiation. I am informed, as he is lowering the gurney upon completion, that today is "doctor" day. I am to wait until Natalie the Nurse calls me to see Dr. Tomlin. Gee, I'm so glad that I was informed of this. What if I had another appointment, or was rushing off to meet someone? I changed into my street clothes and waited. About 10 minutes later, Natalie said, "Jean, let's see the doctor."

On the way down the hall she informed me that we would stop off at the scale as I will be weighed each week. Then she handed me a lab slip and said that I should get my blood drawn today, as they would want to keep track of how my blood count was doing. Great! Another surprise. Dr. Tomlin arrived and asked if I had any questions so far. I did. " What are the sharp "sizzle" pains I feel in my breast?"

"That's normal. It's the nerves regenerating after surgery. You'll most likely feel that for some time." She then asked me to undress.

"Didn't they tell you to stay in your gown until after I had seen you?"

"No one told me about dressing, weighing, lab work or anything. What's the large indentation in my breast from the surgery?

"Well, you had quite a loss of tissue. You probably didn't notice just how much initially because there was so much swelling." Now with the swelling subsided, I have quite a deficit.

Dr. Tomlin then pulled a form from the front of my chart and matter of factly asked, "Would you like to be resuscitated should you need it?" What??? Resuscitated? Was the radiation going to knock me out? As these questions whirled through my mind, I replied, "What is this all about?" She responded that it was a routine form that needed to be signed indicating that should my heart stop while in radiation I would like to be resuscitated. I said that I would and so I signed and Dr. Tomlin witnessed the form. I still couldn't believe that this was such a ho-hum matter, and so I asked if this happened often. She indicated that it did not, but that the technicians needed guidance in case it did. Once again, I was both annoyed and ashamed at this health care system. I assumed that I was a fairly experienced consumer/nurse and yet I was continually surprised at the thoughtlessness.

I then told Dr. Tomlin that we had gone to San Francisco on Monday to see Dr. Kay and that he had given me all the proof I needed to start back on estrogen. Dr. Tomlin looked up from the chart and said, "And what does the oncologist, Dr. Dick say about that?"

"I'm not seeing Dr. Dick any longer. He won't let me talk, or ask questions. And he lied to me about the combined use of estrogen and Tamoxifen." If looks could kill, I would have fallen off the examining table from the blaze of her eyes. After quite a look she said, "Are you willing to see a *woman oncologist?*"

"Where is she located?" "Upstairs, in this building."

"I am willing to see anyone who will talk to me, reason with me, and include me in the plan for MY health." Dr. Tomlin stated that she would make the referral to Dr Katy Rollins. As we left, Gordon asked me why I had even told her about Dr. Kay. Good question, because I could have just let it go and never involved Dr. Tomlin in my decision. I think the reason was a typical patient reaction of wanting

71

to do the right thing, wanting to have the doctor agree with me and, in my case, wanting a coordinated health care team. I was tired of juggling all of these doctors on my own. I really wanted someone to coordinate all of this and then pat me on the head and tell me that I had done everything right. My gosh, I now had seven physicians to deal with and none of them had the total picture of my treatment regimen. Just think if I had a really aggressive cancer, or if I knew nothing about the health care system? I pondered all of this as I headed the car down the street to the lab to have the blood work done.

Day number 5. I finally got my 10:00am time slot. Dakota was back, took me in immediately and I was out in 10 minutes. We were packed, ready to head up the coast. Week one was finished. I'm headed to the beautiful blue ocean...and my estrogen pills.

It was Super Bowl Sunday and we headed down the coast and into the Valley to my son's house to join the family. Well, some of the family as neither of my daughters could attend. But, my sons were present plus two daughters-in-law and three grandchildren. They all told me that I looked terrific. I felt good and we had a wonderful day.

Week number 2, treatment number 6. I followed the instructions, and now had a clean gown since it was Monday. I chose blue, and discovered that it was as big as a tent. Later I found out that a doctor's wife made the gowns from bed sheets. Her patterns must have been very large, but these cloth gowns were much nicer than paper. I was all set and a woman tech came into the room and asked me, "What's your name?" I told her and she said, 'Oh, come on." I followed her into the usual radiation room. She seemed to have problems marking me and getting me set up, but she was friendly and talkative. Well, I reasoned, I guess I get efficient, non-talkative males probing my breast with ink pens, or I get the talkative female who has trouble with the set up. I began to think friendliness might have its price. Finally the linear accelerator started.

Treatment number 7 came with another surprise. I again had Sandra as my technician and she introduced me to yet another female tech that would assist today. Sandra noticed my sports watch and began to ask about it. I really did like the fact that I was noticed; yet the amount of moving the machines, and me and measuring me again and again made me nervous as to why it seemed so difficult today. Then Sandra announced, "Today is x-ray day."

"I don't know anything about."

Sandra said, "Once per week an x-ray is taken to make sure that we are hitting the right spots in the breast."

"How can an x-ray do that?"

"The doctor would explain it on Thursday." Then an x-ray film was *masking taped* to one of the spheres. Now I had masking tape holding up the film (and a warning that I shouldn't jump if it falls off while filming), and a piece of cement in the plastic shield that's secured with a wingnut. I hoped that the actual linear accelerator was shooting those photons at me in a higher tech, more accurate manner.

As I had to wait for a changing room, I returned to the patient's waiting room to find a white haired lady, very bent over at the neck, with a cane by her side and a blanket over her lap. I said hello to her and she returned my greeting with a pleasant smile. We were to become friendly over the next 5 1/2 weeks. But at this point, the patients did not talk to one another.

Day number 8. I arrived confident that I now knew the routine and there would be no more surprises. The two women technicians called me back. "Today is x-ray day," Sandra announced.

"What," I replied. "You did x-rays yesterday."

"Oh, yes, but they didn't turn out right." Great! How much radiation could I tolerate? More questions for the doctor.

Day number 9. It was doctor day again. While waiting today, a pleasant young man (late thirties or early forties) saw that I was reading about "tule fog," which is typical in the central valleys of California. We began talking and he said that he was raised in that area. He was then called in. His name is Alan. I would get to know him better as the weeks unfolded. I noted that he wore a gown for his upper body - as I did. Most of the men were there for prostate and wore the gown to cover a naked lower body. So, I surmised that Alan had an upper body cancer.

Dr. Tomlin explained that the x-rays are required by law to make sure that the parameters of the treatment were correct. The x-ray, however, was only showing rib cage and bones, no soft tissue. Dr. Tomlin was very friendly today telling me that she and her family were coming over to the coast for a weekend visit soon.

Day number 10. Dakota was back as the tech along with the quiet woman from the last two days. They seemed to make a good team. They were fast, efficient and I didn't feel quite as alone. I finished in ten minutes and Gordon and I hit the road for home. Only 5 more weeks to go.

CHAPTER XIII
HYPNOSIS: AN UNEXPECTED ALLY

During the weekend, I received a telephone call from a woman whom I had met at the local Cancer Support Group in November.

"I just started radiation this past week and wondered if we could car pool. I have to leave our coastal town at 8:30 am each morning to arrive at my 12:30 appointment in a town farther south than where you was going." She then had an equally long ride home at the end of the treatment. Twice during that first week, the linear accelerator had broken down prior to her arrival and they could not treat her. One day she just had to turn around and drive home. The second day, they had her wait four hours until the machine was fixed. She felt that her husband, who was the driver, was going to be exhausted and exasperated by the end of seven weeks and she wanted advice. "We got an apartment. Why don't you call the hospital pastoral care unit? I found that she had her surgery in my hospital also. I suggested she call our local Community Resource Connection because they have a van that drives over to the city one day a week. I suggested that she might use that for one day, but strongly encouraged trying to get a place in the treatment city. I could tell she was reluctant, as her husband didn't like to be away from home. I attempted to point out that he was away, at least 8 hours per day at this rate. I realized how wonderful and supportive my husband has been. Gordon treated the move to the city as a "mini" adventure and was willing to go with me.

This woman sounded so down and sad. She had a horrible cold and was trying to stop smoking. She had just bought lots of vitamins that she was going to begin in an attempt to build herself up. "They told me to stop all the antioxidants," I said. She was amazed, as she had not been told this at all.

"You seem so calm and confident about all your treatment" I then told her that I had a "secret weapon" that I was using to get through this time.

"Will you share it with me?"

I told her the following:

I discovered the power of the subconscious mind through hypnosis. It was quite accidental as it related to my cancer. For several months our local newspaper had been running large ads about a certain hypnosis center. The ads were always testimonials from people who said that they had either lost weight or stopped smoking because they had undergone hypnosis therapy. One of the locations was in the city where I was to have the radiation. I have always dieted and am usually trying to lose "the last ten pounds." I had been hypnotized once before during a political campaign when I suddenly started developing a swollen lip every time I had to make a speech. This condition became more and more embarrassing and also more evident to anyone who saw me. A friend who was a psychologist told me that he could hypnotize me and "cure" my lip. I was scared to be hypnotized because I thought that a hypnotized person was out of control and might do something really embarrassing. I had a friend stay in the room with me with the solemn promise that she wouldn't let me do anything embarrassing. What I discovered is that you are not asleep, but only in that dreamy state where your mind is alert but your body is calm and quiet. That one hypnotic suggestion really worked and I have never again had the swollen lip.

Fascinated by the chance to lose 10 pounds while in the city for seven weeks of radiation, I decided to go into the center for a free evaluation. I found a nice group of people and a friendly staff, so I decided to sign up. The next day I had my first appointment with a hypnotist, who asked me, "What is going on in your life." I talked about my recent cancer surgery and my ongoing radiation treatment. I was very surprised that he spent most of the hour and time during the hypnotic session talking about my cancer and what stresses were occurring in my life. The program was organized in such a way that there were classes going on throughout the day on nutrition, psycholinguistics, accelerated learning and group reinforcement sessions. These group classes always concluded with a hypnotic session whereby you heard the suggestions via a headphone connected to a CD. Twice per month each participant had a private session with a hypnotist who recorded the session on an audiotape that you took home and listened to as often as possible. This individual tape was very valuable because it was made just for you after a discussion of what was going on at that point in your life. Several days into the classes I realized that I was getting much more than just nutrition advice. And at the end of the first week, I told the hypnotist that I wanted to heal from the radiation, not burn and that I didn't want to have fatigue. She programmed these thoughts into the tape. I was told that the radiation was healing me and that I was getting stronger and stronger. I was told that my sleep at night would be healing and deep and that I would awaken refreshed and healthy. I listened to the tapes upon awakening in the morning and also at night in bed just before falling to sleep. Of course, I couldn't be sure if any difference was occurring, but I felt good.

Several weeks into my radiation I had two different social functions to attend. At one luncheon, I visited with women who had known me for the past ten years as we had been in tap class twice per week. Everyone told me that I looked great, but it was the telephone call I received the next day that convinced me. One friend called and asked, "What have you done to your face?"

"Why," I asked.

"You look so great - almost as though you have had a face lift - you are glowing." I was delighted. Could this feeling of inner peace really be showing? A few days later I was invited to lunch with two friends from high school. One woman I had not seen in about ten years, the other was Helen, whom I now saw frequently. The two talked after the luncheon. Helen told me that my friend "Couldn't believe how great that you looked." When pushed for specifics she stated that my complexion was radiant and my energy so "bouncy."

But the real proof was going to come during the last weeks when the radiation's cumulative toll would be present. I promised to stay in touch with this other woman who was going to daily radiation. We called each other several times as the weeks rolled by. Each time she had more and more fatigue and by week four her skin had broken down and she had developed weeping small blisters. I developed a rash on my chest and it did get red, but my skin never broke open. By week 6, I did get tired, but only after a full day's activities.

At the last visit with Dr.Tomlin, after I had finished the 33rd treatment, she commented that my skin had come through the treatments better than she ever expected. She also told me that I could experience fatigue for up to a month.

"I am ready to return to aerobics next week."

She told me that would not be wise. Dr.Tomlin suggested that "you might be able to get up to do the dishes or the laundry." Get up? I laughed. Who did she think had been doing the dishes and laundry for the previous seven weeks? As I have talked to others since, I now know that hypnosis allowed me to tap into my subconscious and heal myself. Many people do experience such fatigue that they miss radiation sessions in an attempt to battle the overwhelming tiredness.

The fact that my skin had not broken down allowed me to stay active. Gordon and I walked around several small lakes and trails around the city. I felt better when I could get out and smell the air and experience the sunshine. I wondered why hypnosis was not suggested for people going through cancer treatments. I vowed to discuss this with Dr. Tomlin at some point.

CHAPTER XIV
MY RADIATION "BUDDIES"

Perhaps because I felt so good, or maybe its just the nurse-educator part of my personality, but I wanted to know about the other people whom I saw every day in the patient's waiting room. I wondered if they had come to this place by the same circuitous route as I. We were quite a group when all assembled because the technicians were running late. There was Alan, whom I mentioned earlier. He was still working full-time at a winery where he was in charge of their Chardonnay production. He and his wife had two young boys and had a sixteen-year-old daughter from a previous marriage. Alan and I talked every day for almost a month. I knew all about his goal of producing his own label and the government procedures one must follow. I knew how he lived in the vineyards to allow his sons to run free without worry of cars and busy streets. I knew his hopes and dreams for the future. But, I didn't know what kind of cancer he had! We joked. We laughed. I gave him a "graduation gift" and had a nice note and picture of his family, but I didn't know what kind of cancer he had. I knew the specialist he went to see in San Francisco, I knew the hospital where he was scheduled for chemotherapy for the next several months, but as close as we became, he never once talked about what kind of cancer he had.

Well, Mr. Greeley, who liked to talk, joined us. We all noticed Mr. Greeley for two reasons: he was tall and wore shorts to the radiation office, and he was very outgoing and upbeat. In the beginning.

"Aren't we all lucky to be here?" Mr. Greeley said, by way of a conversation opener.

"Yes," I replied. "I AM very lucky."

But as the weeks wore on, Mr. Greeley felt less and less lucky and more and more fatigued. Although we talked every day, he became more despondent.

"I'm here for prostrate cancer (Did that explain the shorts?). I'm a former marine, and I'll tell you what, never in sam-hell am I putting on one of those sissy print and lace gowns you ladies saddle up in."

Later, he told me about his wife. "She died less than a year ago. Can't seem to take off my wedding ring. You know, she had that diabetes, and the complications had her in a wheel chair for awhile before the end."

He was now very lonely.

"I'd been taking care of her for so long," he said. "I can't get used to being the patient." On Election Day, he told us that he would miss radiation because he was volunteering as a precinct worker at the polls. We cheered him on. The 12-hour day "off" really took it out of him, though, and from then on, he no longer laughed and joked.

One morning I took in a cake. He barely said thank you. "I'm having diarrhea," he said. "I feel drained."

"Have you told your doctor?" I asked, concerned.

"That doctor can't really do anything for me," he replied.

"But you have to ask! And be persistent," I encouraged. At that point, Mr. Greeley turned to Gordon and said, "Your wife has the nicest smile." I wanted to cry out that I would be his friend and his advocate with his doctors forever, but I was suddenly called in to treatment. I did not see Mr. Greeley again. I asked after him with the nurses, they told me he was "taking some time off" to get over his fatigue. I knew he was depressed and withdrawing.

"Will you follow up?"

"Oh, sure, he'll get a call to come back."

Valentine's Day we all arrived to find candy hearts in our "cubbies". How nice and thoughtful. I was encouraged. But, the next day and the day after that I saw that many of the candies were still in front of 50 percent of the cubbies. When I asked Dakota and Gavin, they told me that many patients skipped appointments or "took a vacation" in the middle of their treatments. Why? Some were job or family related, but many were just because the patient needed some time out. Studies have shown, though, that breaking the 6 plus weeks may allow the cancer cells to grow again.

My fellow patients were, for the most part, hanging in there. There was Marion, the white haired, stooped over older lady that I mentioned earlier. Marion was a widow, living in a mobile home park. She had a big choice to make only ten days into her radiation. She had a chance to go on a bus trip with her mobile home group to Reno. Yes, she admitted, it was to gamble, but she did "very little" of that. She got the okay from the doctor and off she went. Upon her return she told us all about the SNOW she had seen for the first time in her life. She described the beauty of the snowflakes as they drifted down to cling on the trees. The trip had obviously made her happy, and she was now ready to see the radiation through to the end. I should mention that both Mr. Greeley and Marion had grown children who transported them to and from their daily appointments. These grownups preferred to wait either in the regular waiting room or in their cars. Some times, they ran errands and returned to pick up their parent.

Connie was probably the most verbal of the group. Dressed in the brightest and most mismatched clothes and worn brown loafers, she would dash into the waiting room, gray tangled braids askew and "plop" into a chair.

"The doctors don't know what they are saying," she said, to no one in particular.

"Why do you say that?" I asked, secretly agreeing with her.

"I've had breast cancer before – thirty years ago. This treatment is excessive for a woman my age. I'm going to be 80 next month, ya know and they tell me I shouldn't walk so much."

Now Connie has the attention of everyone else in the waiting room. Marion puts down her magazine and asks, "HOW old are you?" And "what do you mean, you can't walk?"

Connie then tells us this unbelievable story:

"I'm half Hispanic, half Indian. I have 14 siblings, all dead except one. I married at age 13 and had 11 children."

"I walk because I am afraid to be alone in my apartment. There are too many gangs roaming around and I know that someone will kill me." "You see, my husband was Mexican. We were married for 64 years before he was gunned down by the Mexican Mafia."

By now Connie has us riveted to her story. We are all hoping that we are not called for our radiation treatment. Connie is very thin and quite tall. With her arms wrapped around herself as though to keep her gown from flapping open, she continues:

"My husband was wonderful to me and the kids, but he wasn't always in the best businesses. Ever since he was shot in cold blood in front of our house, I have been nervous to stay alone."

"You live in the same house?" Marion asks, shaking her now not-so-bent white head.

"Oh, no, Connie replies as though talking to a child. "I moved to an apartment, but the tenants are kids and play loud music all the time. So, I walk. I walk all over this city. I walk about nine miles a day. And now they tell me I can't walk here for my appointment."

Not sure whether this women is totally nuts or just misunderstood, I ask "How far do you live from here?"

"Twenty minutes – that's all. And can you believe they send the Cancer Society Van to pick me up and it's always late. So, instead of walking here and arriving on time, I pace back and forth, back and forth and wait. Ridiculous. I'll just stop my treatment and wait for the Mafia to get me."

Practically in unison, the rest of us say, "Oh, Don't do that."

And then Dakota calls me for my radiation. I ask him about Connie and her "wonderfully, rich history."

"Oh, that old gal", he responds, "she's totally nuts."

Oh REALLY? Well, she certainly doesn't fit into the model patient category, and I fear she is going to be written off and not heard at all. She would speak up, but who would respond?

Shirley was a woman with whom I might have become a social friend had we met under different circumstances. When I greeted her on her first day (a 10:30, Monday appointment), she opened up immediately. She was the only woman that had her gown on to protect the lower half of her body. "I have colon cancer, but the operation was botched by a local surgeon." After quite a long period getting diagnosed, she was scheduled to have the cancer removed. Somehow during the surgery, part of the tumor "fell" into the abdominal cavity. When her colon was sewn back together, she was informed that they did not "find" this missing piece. "I went to the University of California Medical Center in San Francisco, and they recommended chemotherapy and radiation for this "remaining piece." She was having the two treatments simultaneously, as her chemotherapy was by mouth (rather than IV as in most cases). " I am very concerned that the radiation will add to my already great fatigue. Did you have chemotherapy?" I'm sure she noted that I had all my hair.

"I didn't have chemotherapy." A handsome man who had joined our group only when the technicians were running late for his appointment spoke up. His name was Don and he was on his last four treatments (boosts).

"I had chemotherapy prior to my radiation and look at my hair." He had a full head of black hair with graying sideburns. He had prostate cancer, and so he and Shirley discussed their "lower body" radiation. The next week, when Donald had his graduation, I took in slices of homemade pastry that a friend had made for me. We all had pastry and coffee as we waited our turn on the linear accelerator.

During the sixth week, I was informed that my appointment the next day would be longer than normal as I was going to be "marked up" for the boosts that would start at the end of that week. I was told that I was scheduled for five boosts not three as I had been told by Dr.Tomlin. The "marking up" procedure was interesting as, once again, any small bit of compassion would have helped. I finished my regular treatment, the machine stopped and the door opened. Instead of the usual okay to take my arm down from its uncomfortable position, Dakota came in and told me to stay in the same position, as the doctor would be in to "mark me up." I waited and waited. Dakota and Gavin left the room, and I could hear them chatting out by the monitors. I squirmed and stared at the little red lights in the ceiling. I read the manufacturers info on the machine, I read the patent number. I was reading ANYTHING to keep from acknowledging how uncomfortable I was. Suddenly Sandra burst into the room, followed by Dakota and Gavin, and said, "Oh, Jean, put your arm down and let's cover you up. The doctor is on a long distance call and won't be here for a few more minutes." At which point Gavin asked me, "Would you like a blanket?" Where had they been for the last ten minutes? And I wondered how Connie or Marion handled the same, unfeeling, dispassionate care?

Dr. Tomlin arrived with an x-ray that she placed over my breast as a guide and then made an outline with the proverbial green felt pen. That was to be the total area covered by the boost that would be delivered on "the other accelerator, in the other room." After she left, Dakota went over the green felt with a thicker blue pen and told me not to wash it off. Three days later then, I was ushered into the "other room." There I found a much newer linear accelerator with a narrow arm which came down to within a couple of inches of the marked breast. Attached to this arm was a cut out of the same design as was outlined on my breast. The technicians were women; one I had seen before and the other new to me. They explained, "The shields are in the machine and you will now get an electron beam that is more shallow and specific. You were getting photons that go deeper and wider." However, to get into position for this treatment I had to turn on my left side pull my knees up and put my right arm up and over my forehead. There was no plastic arm guard, the gurney was very narrow and the position was difficult to hold without moving. When the technicians left the room, I could not only hear the machine trying to start, but also could see little tabs on the arm going back and forth. After several tries, the tech was back. "Something is wrong with your position," she stated. I asked about the clicking noise and she said that was the accelerator trying to start but being stopped because the computer coordinates didn't match up. She allowed as how she had tried to "override" the machine but it wouldn't work. "I'm sorry." I hastened to say "I can stand anything as long as the electrons are hitting the correct target." I moved my arm into a better position on the pillow that stuck out from the top of my head and that position seemed to work. The next attempt and the machine whirled away, but for only 30 seconds. The boost was over for day one!

Mary joined the waiting room on my last week. Wearing a baseball cap and a gown, that covered a naked torso from the waist up, I surmised that she was a breast cancer patient.

"I am. How long have you been coming for radiation?" When I told her, she asked me about skin care.

"I brought a bottle of aloe vera gel into my cubbie and use it after each treatment" She looked shocked. "I can't believe that you can leave it in the cubbie. They told me to use the gel when I got home." But as she went back to work, she hadn't been using it.

"My skin is in good shape, just a tan under my armpit. I have a bottle of gel at home and one in my cubbie. The gel is colorless and odorless and doesn't stain clothing. It is perfect and soothing. I apply it several times a day, but always after my shower, after my radiation and before going to bed." On my very last day, as I was dressed and ready to leave, Mary took me aside and showed me her tube of gel - in the back of her cubbie. "Why don't they tell patients to have their gel in their cubbie?" she asked. "I don't know, but you tell every patient that you meet in the waiting room." You carry the message from here on.

After that last appointment, I had the usual appointment with Dr. Tomlin. I was weighed in and congratulated by an ever-enthusiastic Natalie the Nurse. "Wow, your skin looks terrific - -no burning. And you didn't miss one appointment due to fatigue. How did you do this?"

"Hypnosis," I answered.

"Really? You'll have to tell Dr. Tomlin about that."

Dr. Tomlin had the same exclamation when I gave her the same answer. I then spent some time explaining the value of hypnosis to me. "Why don't you refer patients undergoing radiation to some mind-body connection resource?"

Her only answer was based upon the cost, which was an unknown to her. "How did you find Positive Changes and what were the costs, the benefits."

"I promise to get you more information." I believe that, while physicians in general might be vaguely interested, they do not know much about the great resource of the patient's own subconscious in the healing process. This is not taught in medical school and now they are busy with careers and not really interested in learning a new modality. Maybe I'm being too critical, but that is my impression. If only the health care profession would embrace the ability of the patient to be a part of the healing process, what changes could be accomplished? The mind, whether in the form of prayer, meditation or hypnosis, is a powerful tool and right along with medicine, surgery and radiation could affect the outcome for cancer patients.

I had but two other comments and questions for Dr. Tomlin and these were concerning the delivery of care.

"Why," I asked "do the women technicians take care of the mostly male population receiving radiation and the men technicians treat the mostly female populations on the large linear accelerator?"

The answer was incredible!

"Well," she replied. "It has to do with weight. You see, the larger, older machine has plastic shields on the two spheres with the hunk of cement secured with a wingnut. These weights have to be put into place for each individual patient and then removed and put back on the shelf before the next patient is seen. The weights are between one and two pounds and with the number of patients seen per day, that is a great deal of lifting. The newer linear accelerator has internal guards so there is no lifting of these weights."

Dr Tomlin smiled at me as though her explanation was crystal clear and sufficient.

I was aghast!

"You mean that these young vigorous technicians can't lift a couple of pounds of weight about thirty to forty times per day? What about a mother of a toddler or pre-schooler who lifts kids in and out of equipment all day long, seven days per week?"

Dr Tomlin just smiled her usual pleasant, quiet smile and waited for me to change the subject. Week and months later, I am still puzzled at this logic that considers only the convenience of the employees and totally disregards the feelings of the patients.

I then asked about my second concern.

"After six weeks or so, the folks who arrive in the waiting room every day become familiar with each other. It seems to me that this would be a great time for education and dialogue. My little group had begun to chat about skin changes, and even bodily functions. As an old nurse-educator, I think this would be a great place, for say a volunteer nurse, to help out by informally chatting with each group."

"Oh, we have considered an idea," she answered enthusiastically. "We thought that we could get a retired Seeing Eye Dog for the waiting room --you know, for the patients to pet." As my eyes grew wider and my mouth fell open, she added, "Older patients need tactile stimulation."

"WE'RE NOT BLIND," my mind shouted, "We have CANCER!"

The closing of my chart indicated that my time was up and the appointment was over. This was as far as it was to go. I would organize some volunteers myself, but I live two hours away. Instead I write this experience in the hopes that it will help others facing breast cancer treatment choices.

CHAPTER XV
HORMONE REPLACEMENT THERAPY?
THE ANSWER?
OR
THE PROBLEM?

Nothing in this world seems to remain constant for very long. It reminds me of the old sixties soap opera, "As the World Turns," that opened with a picture of the globe slowly revolving. And so it was that after sleeping well and feeling terrific for six months, attributing it all to my low dose 0.5mg of estrogen, that the headlines screamed, *Drug Trial Ordered Stopped.* That was followed by the Los Angeles Times story, *Long-term estrogen use linked to rise in ovarian cancer risk.* Reading the stories very carefully, it became apparent that the drug trial by the Women's Health Initiative of the National Heart, Lung and Blood Institute was very credible. It had enrolled more than 16,000 women between the ages of 50 and 79 who had not had a hysterectomy or history of heart disease. The study ran for five years, and had an additional three years to go, before being abruptly halted after finding that the risks for heart attacks, strokes, breast cancer and blood clots had exceeded a previously determined threshold of acceptability. However, the number of cases of colorectal cancer and hip fractures were less than expected. The number of endometrial cancers and deaths remained what researchers call "neutral."

My first reaction was, "Oh, no, just when I had this figured out." But, I began to read more carefully and specifically. The headlines and first few paragraphs talked only of estrogen. It was not until I read the very last paragraphs that I found that the women in a parallel study, who had hysterectomies, and were, therefore only on estrogen, were continuing on the drug. What was going on here? I logged onto my computer and found the basic Women's Health Initiative Study and read the entire story from the source. I discovered that the drug that had been stopped, was a combination drug containing both estrogen and progesterone. The progesterone is the hormone produced in the second half of the menstrual cycle and is given to post-menopausal women in order to prevent the buildup of estrogen in the uterus. I decided to review the basic physiology.

During a woman's childbearing years, she has two major reproductive hormones working each month. Estrogen begins to build during the first days of the cycle because it stimulates the ovaries to produce and then release an egg. At the point of this release, or ovulation, the second major hormone, progesterone begins to build. Progesterone is a powerful drug. It is responsible for maintaining the healthy lining of the uterus preparing it to receive the fertilized egg. After the progesterone level is high, if there is no fertilized egg, the hormone level drops and menstruation occurs. It is this build up of progesterone that causes the typical PMS (premenstrual syndrome) symptoms of water retention, headaches, and emotional upsets that many women experience for a week or so prior to the menstrual period.

In preparing drugs for post-menopausal women, scientists had found that they needed to use both estrogen and progesterone. This finding had occurred many years ago, when the use of estrogen alone was linked to increased uterine cancer. It was found that if the uterus had a continual buildup of estrogen, without menstrual cleansing caused by the action of progesterone, cancerous changes might occur. Hence, it made sense to replicate a woman's normal menstrual cycle during menopause. However, most post-menopausal women didn't really want to continue bleeding every month. Having endured years of pads and tampons, who wanted that in their "golden years?"

Science responded again by producing a low dose progesterone that could be taken every day of the month - just enough to prevent the estrogen buildup, but low enough to prevent the unpleasant pseudo menstrual period every month. Then one further step took place. Why not combine the two drugs, estrogen and the low dose progesterone into one, easy to take drug? Why not indeed. And so Wyeth Pharmaceuticals manufactured a drug named Prempro.. The relief from menopausal symptoms was well documented, and by the year 2001 there were 22.3 million prescriptions written for this drug

Only at the very end of most articles about the Women's Health Initiative Study was there a line or two stating that women who were on the estrogen only study would continue taking estrogen. Wait a minute. Read that over again!

"Researchers stress that another part of the study, involving postmenopausal women who have had hysterectomies and are taking the estrogen-only drug, Premarin, is continuing." So, what do we

conclude? I decided that the message was that progesterone might be the real culprit and not the estrogen. I re-read what Dr. Kay had told me. He said to use progesterone sparingly -- every few months to clean out the uterus, but not on a continuous basis. And that I was to use a high dose (5mg) for fourteen days, replicating a regular menstrual cycle. He also had told me that I should have a "normal period" after completing the drug. Dr. Kay had given me the option of taking progesterone every two, three or four months depending upon how productive the flow. He stated that progesterone should only be used to ensure that the buildup of estrogen in my uterus was not too great. He suspected that the continuous progesterone could have caused the few fibroids that I was developing. I recalled how I had started bleeding when I was on continuous progesterone even though it was not combined with my estrogen. Within two months of the onset of that bleeding, my breast lump had been discovered. I remembered that I had been on this low dose progesterone drug for about eight years. Coincidence? Or could it be that progesterone was the real problem, and not the estrogen?

I went back to my computer where I logged into the Journal of the American Medical Association. I downloaded the entire 23 pages on, *Risks and Benefits of Estrogen Plus Progestin in Healthy Postmenopausal Women. Principal results from the Women's Health Initiative Randomized Controlled Trial* and started reading very carefully. On page 12, I found the following two paragraphs under: "Limitations."

"This trial tested only 1 drug regimen, CEE, 0.625mg/d, plus MPA, 2.5 mg/d, in postmenopausal women with an intact uterus. The results do not necessarily apply to lower dosages of these drugs, to other formulations of oral estrogens and progestins, or to estrogens and progestins administered through the transdermal route. It remains possible that transdermal estradiol with progesterone which more closely mimics the normal physiology and metabolism of endogenous sex hormones may provide a different risk-benefit profile."

"Importantly, this trial could not distinguish the effects of estrogen from those of progestin. The effects of progestin may be important for breast cancer and atheroscerotic diseases, including CHD and stroke. Per protocol, in a separate and adequately powered trial, WHI is testing the hypothesis of whether oral estrogen will prevent CHD in 10,739 women who have had a hysterectomy............At an average follow-up of 5.2 years, the DSMB has recommended that this trial continue because the balance of overall risks and benefits remains uncertain. These results are expected to be available in 2005 at the planned termination." [1]

So, there it was: one type of combined estrogen and progesterone has caused a slight risk. Slight is specifically that for every 10,000 women taking this drug, eight more would have breast cancer than the women taking nothing. And that is for only one type of combined drug. We have just seen that other combinations are unknown. And, the study where women are only taking estrogen continues. Amazing what happens when you dissect the headlines and carefully read the entire research study.

I feel wonderful again. I believe that pouring through this lengthy document has relieved my concern about my decision. How would others feel?

I belong to two separate small groups of women. Both groups just happened to meet within a week after the alarming headlines about HRT. All of the women, about fifteen in number, are postmenopausal. Some have been on hormones for years. Others have been on and off and a few have never taken any replacement hormones. Fear and concern were paramount during both meetings. Several had quit their HRT immediately and feared the return of hot flashes. Others had made appointments to see their physicians. In fact, I was the only one who stated that I was going to continue on my daily low dose (0.5 mg) of estrogen and my once every four months dose of progesterone. What became very apparent was that these women were reacting to the news stories, and not to the facts. One member is a physician and she and I tried to educate our friends on the two hormones, estrogen and progesterone. But all the women could hear was that estrogen equals increased risk for breast cancer, heart disease, stroke and blood clots. We found that one woman, with no uterus, was on progesterone plus estrogen. We encouraged her to question the reason for this with her physician. Another woman had used the transdermal patch successfully for years and yet could not be consoled by my report that no problems had been found with that method of transmission. These smart, educated women who had been in take-charge careers were suddenly willing to follow incomplete reporting in the local newspaper. Pointing out the need to really understand what type of HRT they were on did no good. And no one wanted to read the journal report that I offered. They believed that their own doctors would know what was best and would tell them – almost without them asking.

Three months later, I asked each of these same women to send me an email describing what hormones they had taken in the past and what they had changed after the news reports that summer. All of the women who were previously on hormones had made some changes! Some had merely gone to lower doses of estrogen and a couple of women had switched to vaginal estrogen preparations only. Four women just stopped taking their HRT on the day the news reported that the hormone study was halted. Of those four, one has gone back on her HRT after having a significant recurrence of symptoms like night sweats, sleep disruption, and hot flashes. The other three have remained off of any hormones, but have menopausal symptoms again. Each of them thinks that they can weather this period and permanently stay off. The one woman who was taking a combined dose although she had no uterus has elected to stay with estrogen only with the hope of discontinuing it gradually. The woman who had been on HRT the longest, about 25 years, has switched to a natural progesterone and vaginal estrogen. All of the women hope that they can maintain their new regimen.

I found that my friends mirrored the response by the post-menopausal women of the country when a *New York Times* article on

November 10, 2002 reported similar findings. [2] Data is difficult to collect, but the one figure that speaks loudly is the one showing that the sales of Prempro are down from 2.7 million to 1.5 million. Anecdotal stories abound. Some women just quit their hormones and although suffering hot flashes and night sweats have determined to ride it out. Others will go so far as to use a long dose estrogen vaginal cream to counteract the vaginal dryness that makes sex painful and libido a distant memory. Others, such as Iretta Taylor, a customer service adviser in Houston, Texas, told the *New York Times* journalist that she tried to live without hormone therapy but decided she would rather not. Mrs. Taylor, age 49 explained:

"I went into menopause at a very early age, at about 40, and it was a very bad, very emotional time. I was edgy, depressed; I thought I was having a nervous breakdown. I had hot flashes, too and a hollow, dry look and dryness in the vaginal area, which was no fun."

"As soon as I started taking HRT, it all went away," she said, referring to hormone therapy by its old name, H.R.T. for hormone replacement therapy. A co-worker told me, 'Your skin looks so fine'

It did; I had a real glow.

"When I head all the horror stories last summer I stopped," she said. " I didn't even call my doctor; I just stopped. Right away I started to feel bad again. I thought at first that it was psychosomatic, but then I realized, 'Honey, it's the hormones.'

"I asked my doctor, 'Please put me back on H.R.T.' and he did. Now, she said, I feel like a woman is supposed to feel. If they ban this

in the United States, I'll drive down to Mexico to get it. That's how much I need my H.R.T." [3]

The real question, then, is this: Is Mrs.Taylor typical of most women or is she quite unusual? No one seems to know. The women who have severe symptoms seem to be driven to seek prescriptions for hormone replacement therapy of some type. How many women just suffer in silence or don't really suffer at all is still unknown.

Many of the doctors quoted in the various news articles since July state that women are too swept up in a desire to remain youthful. Several state that fifty-year-old women should just realize that at fifty, one does not look or feel thirty. Women need to be comfortable with how they look and feel, no matter what the their age. Again, it is a matter of making a personal decision. There is no right or wrong way; no black or white.

And what about Alzheimer's disease? There has only been cursory information that taking estrogen would protect the brain. My own experience with my mother's Alzheimer's disease has made this estrogen to brain relationship hypothesis paramount for me. My mother was never on hormone replacement therapy, and at age seventy-eight developed Alzheimer's. On the other hand, her older sister, now over one hundred years old, who also never took HRT, is alive, well and mentally sound. The jury is out on this one. Researchers express opinions on both sides of the question of estrogen intake and memory. Some feel that if estrogen is taken for a prolonged period, memory loss is minimized or prevented. But there is agreement on the fact that no large study has been done in this area.

Some scientists purport that this is the time to do a study since there is no preventative drug for Alzheimer's. A study, using sufficient numbers of women, would be very helpful.

I was asked by some of my friends what I thought that they should do. I offered my opinion based upon my research and encouraged them to see their health provider. I was surprised that some just really wanted me tell them what to ask and what to say. How could the medical profession have such a terrifying grip on these intelligent women? Knowledge is power, and I encouraged them to put in the time and research to take control of their own bodies. Some admitted to concern regarding wrinkles, night sweats and reduced libido, but also stated that their doctors would consider these concerns trivial. I would hope that any woman could talk about her concerns with her physician, and if treated without respect or concern, immediately change doctors.

The media continues to carry stories about the Women's Health Initiative Study. Now these articles speak about what women are taking in order to feel good, but hopefully without the risks of estrogen. Words like "natural" and "plant-based" are utilized to convey that women can still have a safe estrogen supply. As one writer commented, she wouldn't mind looking eighty years old, but she didn't want to look sixty. Somehow, society condones gray hair and wrinkles at eighty, but not at sixty.

What to do? Evaluate your own risk factors. Do you have a family history of heart disease, stroke, breast or colon cancer? Take osteoporosis and Alzheimer's into consideration. Put all of these conditions into your own health equation along with how you feel and how you want to feel. If you can write these down, then you can share them with your health care provider. Together then, you can devise a plan that takes into consideration how you want to feel and what level of risk you are willing to take. No two women are exactly alike and we should not, therefore, compare ourselves to what our friends are taking or not taking. Know your own body and mind and do what is best for you, emotionally, mentally and physically. By the time this ink is dry, there will be new studies and new theories. By understanding your own risk factors, you will be able to maintain your quality of life goal.

CHAPTER XVI
THE VALUE OF YOUR SUPPORT SYSTEM

The entire breast cancer experience doesn't happen in a vacuum, and so must necessarily include those closest to the patient. My situation was no different, and I have been asked how my husband felt, acted and reacted throughout the acute phases of my seven-month treatment period.

When coming out of his anesthesia from hand surgery, Gordon remembered that I was across the street at the Imaging Center having my annual mammogram. But, he remembered how frightened we had both been in 1990 when we had received the call about my first abnormal mammogram. He opened his eyes to see me standing at his bedside and when he asked about the mammogram, I responded by saying that we would talk about it later. As the anesthesia worked its way out of his system, Gordon was groggy and falling asleep after repeatedly asking the same question. During the two-hour ride home we laughed about the repeated question. But, once at home and with a little soup in his stomach, I explained that a small mass had been found and that I was scheduled for a needle biopsy the following week. We decided that the best thing to do was act normally, since we had a plan. It was, perhaps, easier for me to concentrate on his recovering fingers, because I needed to help change dressings and apply and reapply his splint each day.

Due to the timing of the biopsy, Gordon was in his first hand therapy session and could not be with me. But, he had the staff notify me when he arrived at the Imaging Center. The room was so tiny that he could not have been present even if he had not a conflicting appointment. But, it was comforting to know that he would be there when I was finished.

During the two-hour ride home, we discussed the procedure and the fact that in twenty-four hours we would have an answer. Gordon said, "We're moving forward. We can deal with most anything except ignorance." I know that Gordon has always assumed that because of our almost fifteen year age difference, he would be the first to die. I think that that has always been a comforting thought for him, and one that he firmly believes will be played out. Therefore, it was not going to be a terminal situation that we faced, at least not in his mind.

During the call from Dr. Poojoolian, Gordon was downstairs in his study. When the biopsy report was read to me and I started asking questions about whether or not we should proceed with a planned trip, Gordon came upstairs to be with me when the conversation ended. I was very scattered in my thinking and needed to leave for a scheduled meeting with my circle of women. Gordon encouraged me to ask for advice. Upon my return 3 hours later, I had cried, talked to my son and was ready to plan how to proceed. Gordon totally supported my request for a second opinion. He was willing to pay out of pocket if our insurance would not pay for the second opinion, but encouraged me to talk to our local doctor first.

When we began to make visits to the oncologist and the surgeon, Gordon always accompanied me. In all instances the office staff invited him to join me in the examining and consultation rooms. I would have walked out if they had tried to keep him away! However, there was a great difference once we were in the doctor's office. Dr. Dick, the medical oncologist, spoke directly to Gordon. We were seated side by side. I was the one with all the questions. And yet the doctor maintained more eye contact with Gordon than with me. Especially on the second visit, after my surgery, I was told to "not ask questions, until I'm finished." I think the doctor was hoping that Gordon would persuade me to take chemotherapy, the treatment that Dr. Dick pushed that day.

In fact, the only time that I felt insensitivity from Gordon was after we left Dr. Dick' office. It was noon and Gordon asked where I wanted to go for lunch. When I started crying, he realized that food was not my concern at that moment. He did not seem to understand how undone I was at arguing with the doctor and, of course, secretly wondering if I was wrong. He really thinks I'm tougher than I am. After lunch, where I talked and talked, we needed to proceed on to the appointment with the surgeon. Gordon did have me stop at a grocery store so that he could run in for some items for dinner. I should state here that I do the driving and Gordon does the cooking and that arrangement works very well for us. Gordon hates driving, and I did enough cooking while raising my five children. Gordon is a gourmet cook, but at times his need for ingredients can be awkward. This was one of those times. I grabbed by cell phone and called two of my circle members. Neither was available, so I poured out my sorrows on the phone. Neither answering machine cared what I said. I felt better.

Shortly after, we approached the surgeon's office, only to be hit by a truck. I was pulling into a diagonal parking spot and the truck was leaving rapidly. The driver turned too sharply and bang; he hit the right rear section of our station wagon. I was completely undone. Gordon handled everything. He talked to the driver, got his insurance, called our insurance, and even set up the time to have the car checked after the appointment. Luckily for me, my youngest daughter, Lorna, was meeting me there and she literally rubbed my back and let me talk out my fears.

Maybe it was Gordon's faith in God that helped him get through my two separate surgeries. He was with me until I was wheeled into the operating room and came to see me as soon as he was permitted. I too have great faith and I was not afraid. I was glad to have both Gordon and God on my side.

The toughest part for me was wondering about my new, small, disfigured breast. When the first bandage came off, I had my daughter-in-law, the registered nurse, help me remove the tape. Later, after a shower, I showed Gordon and he just said, "I love you, not the shape of your breast." While I knew that in my heart, it was very nice to hear those words. After the second surgery where a second golf ball size mass of tissue was removed, the breast deficit was even more noticeable. Worse, for me, is the fact that the suture pulls the nipple up and over to the right. I feel as though I have a nipple pointing under my armpit, while my other nipple points somewhat south from too many children combined with aging. Gordon encouraged me to do whatever would make me feel good about myself - be it a padded bra, corrective surgery or whatever. I hate to shop and when in the city, I said, "Oh, its too late to get a new bra."

Gordon said, "Take your time and do it." As a proverbial hater of shops and shopping, this was just the push that I needed. I guess I wanted him to care about how I looked and needed that reassurance.

Even now, one year later, I still hate the way that breast looks. The radiation has caused the nipple and areola to be faded and light pink in color. My other breast is more robust and darker in color. I pointed this out to Gordon. "Yea, Jean. But who will know that? Who's going to care?" Indeed, I'm not planning on going topless. Gordon shows love, and I think, is comfortable with my appearance. He states that even a mastectomy, if that had been my choice, would not have made any difference in his feelings for me.

Radiation caused us to uproot our residence for 7 weeks. I think Gordon found that more difficult than my surgery. Gordon is a "control" kind of man and for seven weeks we were going to live in a small, furnished apartment in a strange town. We would only have our lap top computer and our cell phone. At first, we treated the experience as a grand experiment. We enjoyed eating out, hiking around the various lakes and rivers and catching up on movies. But, several weeks into our stay, Gordon suggested, "Maybe I'll stay home next week and get things done." I was very hurt. I was going to my first appointment with Dr. Rollins and he wouldn't be there. I didn't want to ask as I am very capable of handling appointments on my own, but it was just emotional support that would be missing. My circle of women was going to drive the two hours to my apartment to have our Thursday meeting, and I was truly touched and moved that they would do this. Gordon felt that this justified his remaining home since, if the group came for the two-hour meeting, he would have to leave.

Although I filled my days with friends and dinner one night with my brother and sister-in-law, I felt deserted. Then on the Thursday morning, many of the circle could not make the trip and the meeting was cancelled. I frantically called Gordon to please get a ride to town. He immediately called some good friends who made the trip over to the city, met me for lunch, and I was happy once again. I think that Gordon felt badly when he realized that I had been upset. But with now only two weeks left, he decided to take a train trip to the central part of the state to visit his ailing sister. I could understand the logic of the trip, but again felt that I was being left because my day-in-day-out radiation was becoming very boring. Taking Gordon to the train necessitated a long drive for me down and back to the station on busy, congested freeways. He agreed to take a bus back to the "radiation" city on his return. Gordon also visited his newly engaged son, and took him and his fiancée out to dinner. In these last two weeks, I think that Gordon was no longer concerned that I was having any problems, and it was just a matter of the daily radiation until the end of the seventh week.

Gordon has always deferred to me on the question of whether or not to continue taking estrogen. He has questioned me, and I think would truly like me to stop. However, he is willing to read anything that I suggest on the subject and believes it is my body and therefore my choice. I don't mind defending my choice and rather enjoy our discussions of same.

Gordon is not an overly demonstrative person but he is logical, loyal and loving. He is easily bored by both repetition and redundancy. He loves me and I have no fear of losing his love. I would be concerned, however, if I was ever in a nursing home where routine was the key. Gordon hates routine. But that's another story.

CHAPTER XVII
MY HUSBAND:
IN HIS OWN WORDS!

This is Jean's story. But after a male friend of ours read the first few chapters of her book, he asked, "What did your husband think about and how did he feel during the ordeal? I would wonder about my emotions if this should happen to my wife." After some thought, Jean asked me to add a few words about my perspective during her adventure.

Cancer is a scary word. Since her first surgery 11 years earlier for the pre-cancerous breast condition, I felt a sense of dread every time she made an appointment for a mammogram. The fact that this DCIS would become invasive decreased as time went on. But, I remember how frightened we had both been in 1990 when the call came about her first abnormal mammogram. I couldn't shake the feeling that our luck would run out; and that maybe this time we would get bad news and she indeed had cancer.

Each time she went for testing I prayed. We don't expect our faith in God to preclude problems. We have learned, though, that He gives us the strength to face any tribulation when it arises.

As I came out of the fog of anesthesia following my hand surgery, I remembered that she was across the street at the Imaging Center, having her annual mammogram. I recall opening my eyes to see Jean standing at my bedside. My first words were to ask about the mammogram. When she didn't directly answer to tell me that the results were negative, I knew that the news was cancer.

As the anesthesia worked its way out of my system, I was still groggy and kept falling asleep after asking the same question. During the two-hour ride home, we actually began laughing about the constant repetition. When we arrived home and she gave me soup, she told me that a small mass had been found and that she was scheduled for a needle biopsy on the following week.

In a sense, I was calmed. There is no fear worse than that of the unknown. At least now we could plan action. However, until the report came back indicating a problem, the best thing to do was act normally. It was easier for us to concentrate on my recovering fingers, since Jean needed to change dressings and apply and reapply my splint each day.

After she had the biopsy we discussed the procedure and the fact that in twenty-four hours we would have an answer. I felt so grateful that I could be with her and that we were moving forward. We could deal with most anything except ignorance and uncertainty.

Because I am almost fifteen years older than my wife I had subconsciously always assumed that I would be the first to die. I had read all the books and articles focusing on "Teaching Your Wife To Be A Widow." And indeed, the wills and family trust and were set up so that she would face a minimum of distress. But now, the thought, "What would I do without Jean?" kept jumping into my head. I pushed that thinking out of my mind. I focused on the hope that this wasn't a terminal situation, but only an unpleasant period of surgery that she faced.

When Dr. Poojoolian phoned the next day, I was downstairs in my study. I could clearly hear Jean's side of the conversation. After the biopsy report was read to her, she started asking questions about whether or not we should proceed with a planned trip. I came upstairs to be with her when the conversation ended. We were both rather scattered in our thinking. Jean needed to leave for a scheduled meeting with her "circle" of women. Even though I wanted to be with her and discuss our options, I was relieved that I would not be the only one listening to her fears regarding the next steps. I encouraged her to ask for their advice. When she returned 3 hours later she said that it had been helpful to share her emotions and concerns with other women. She then phoned her children and was ready to plan our next step. .

I have always been pleased that Jean knows her way around the medical system. We both felt that a second opinion was a logical course of action. If our insurance wouldn't pay for this, I was willing to pay out of pocket. However, I encouraged her to talk to our local doctors first.

Of course I accompanied Jean on the visits to the oncologist and the surgeon. In each instance the receptionist invited me to join her in the examining and consultation rooms. However, it was interesting to see the difference between the two doctors once we were in the privacy of their office. Although the surgeon, Dr. Sweet, was gracious toward me and willingly answered my concerns, her focus was always on the patient--Jean. Dr. Dick, the medical oncologist, maintained eye contact only with me and rarely spoke directly to Jean. She had most of the questions. Yet even when he answered her he would give her a brief glance, respond to her inquiry but all the while looking at me while he answered. It was very strange.

And then she had the surgery to remove the cancer. In the days leading up to the procedure it was easy for me to focus on giving her emotional support. I didn't have a chance to think of myself. But as I sat in the waiting room during the operation the old question, "What would I do without her?" returned. It was only with great effort that I was able to push these fears out of my mind. We were, after all, following a logical procedure. I assured myself that the results would be positive. Jean was so brave and so upbeat that I told myself that the least I do was to mirror her courage. Still it was tough keeping the fears out of my mind.

After Jean's recovery from the surgery, she returned to Dr. Dick for her follow-up. His failure to talk directly to her was as noticeable as before. When she, understandably started the conversation with a query, he interrupted with "Please don't ask questions until I'm finished." He complacently proceeded to outline on a sheet of paper the treatment she "would" follow. As he wrote he said, "You will, of course, have chemotherapy." When she tried to interject questions about side effects, he again said, "Please wait until I have finished." After he had finished his dicta, he looked at me and said, "Now, do you have any questions?" Jean then asked about contraindications to chemotherapy and side effects. He verbally dismissed her concerns as irrelevant as he continued to look at me. When she said that she would consider the suggestions, he seemed nonplussed and said to me, "I strongly urge you to follow my treatment procedure." Did he think that I was the only one making decisions about her health?

Were there some relationships where the wife deferred to her husband and the doctor about her health? This might be true in some marriages, but certainly not ours. Did he think that I would persuade her to take this treatment over her objections? Maybe he thought that I could order her to do so. I became so irritated by his attitude that I failed to focus on what his words were doing to my wife.

Because we were seated side by side, I could only hear her voice and didn't see the anguish on her face. Because I was confused by Dr. Dick, I failed to notice her need for support as she made a difficult decision. I'm afraid that as close as we are, during her surgery and treatment I often failed to appreciate her emotions. As we left his office she began to cry -- one of the few times in our marriage. I then realized my error. Jean is a marvelous, bright, strong and incisive woman. Sometimes I think that she is tougher than she is.

To make a difficult day even more emotional, as we were parking for the appointment with the surgeon; a truck hit our car. This wasn't a good day. I'm just glad that I was there to take care of the accident details while she kept the date with Dr. Sweet. Luckily her younger daughter was meeting us at the office. Lorna rubbed her back, let her talk out her fears and gave extra comforting. Sometimes it is easier for me to handle "things" than to soothe.

Jean's radiation was, to me, a mixed bag of experiences and emotions. The challenge of coping in a small apartment in an unfamiliar town, the daily visits for radiation and seeing so many sad patients, the joy of being with my wife as we explored a new city, the reaffirmation of Jean's courage and our love--all these took place.

Jean told me that one of the toughest emotions was her concern over how I would react to her post-surgical breast. Although it didn't occur to me at the time, I guess this was predictable. Adolescent "guy" talk and glossy advertising both focus on the breast as essential to female beauty and sexual desirability.

When I was a teenager, I probably felt that way about women. But we have had a wonderful life together, including a fulfilling sexual relationship. To my eye, Jean's loveliness is so much greater than that of other women that it transcends physical beauty. And, a smile and a twinkle in her eye are the most sexually exciting stimulus I can imagine. I honestly didn't feel those post-surgical scars or even (had it been necessary) mastectomy would have had an effect on my vision of her. Beauty really isn't only in the eye of the beholder. When a person really loves, the beauty is in his memory and his heart. I don't think that I'm very different than most men in this regard.

I was asked how I felt about the therapy she chose. Would I have been happier if she had followed conventional medical treatment and had chemotherapy? I believe that people have right to make decisions about their own body. I always defer to Jean on questions of her treatment. As much as I love her, it is her body and therefore her choice. I am willing to read anything on treatment, and see my role as her partner to support the decision she makes.

I only keep my right to question her decision before the fact and then support her afterwards without reservation.

Jean and I share a deep faith in a loving and personal God. This has certainly helped both of us through this ordeal. This isn't a subject that is easy for me to discuss. But I am sure that we would not have been so blessed in the results of her treatment if we had not turned to the Almighty for aid.

CHAPTER XVIII
WHERE DO WE GO FROM HERE?
CONCLUSIONS

This book could go on forever, as the final chapters are not yet written. Just today my mailbox contained a respected university health newsletter. It contained an article titled, "Postmenopausal hormones: Where do we go from here?" [4] One of its concluding sub-headings is "Could it be the Progestin?" [5] And so, the quest for the culprit continues.

Throughout my experience and certainly since I have been writing, I have spoken with many women who are worried about breast cancer, have had breast cancer or have just been diagnosed. I have participated in groups with fellow cancer survivors and some who thought they had survived only to have discover that it was only a remission. It is so easy to get caught up in the fervor of diagnosis and treatment that you to lose sight of the long-term goal. And that goal is to live your life on your terms! Sure, a dreadful diagnosis might be handed to you. But, your worst fears are usually your imagined fears. Getting fears spelled out and questions answered are the best ways to proceed. Knowledge gives us the power to make decisions that our right for us. Breast cancer is usually a slow growing cancer and you don't need to feel that you must make immediate decisions about how to proceed.

My biggest mistake was when I rushed into having the second surgery instead of waiting until Dr. Logan returned in seven days. Imagine, I could have saved myself an entire surgery if I had just waited a few more days. So, take your time, investigate, ask questions and above all, feel comfortable about the decisions you make --for the decisions are yours and yours alone.

The lessons that I learned and would share are summed up as follows:

There is no one correct method of treatment for any breast cancer.

It is your right and responsibility to research and question all options for care offered to you.

Always get a second opinion - it is worth every penny for your peace of mind.

Request a copy of every test done before, during and after your diagnosis and treatment.

Start and maintain a complete file of all your health data. It is your right, and your responsibility to collect and hold all the information on your health. Most times these copies are given with a smile and no charge. Occasionally, with a growl and a charge. Either way, you need a copy of all your reports for your file. Then you are ready to seek better advice as to your care and ultimately to make more accurate decisions.

- ◆ Ask where you can verify information given to you, i.e. the internet, health journals, the library.
- ◆ Health care is changing and improving constantly so make sure that you are not getting outdated or old advice.

119

◆ Take the time to visualize what kind of outcome you wish to have. What in life is important to you? Do not be rushed to make a decision. After all, the breast cancer took some time to grow. It did not happen overnight.

◆ Request the procedures that are best for you: biopsy, surgery, medication, rehabilitation, hypnosis, whatever it is.

◆ Be ready to change doctors if your voice is not heard and respected.

◆ Don't just "go along" to be a good patient. A good patient could be a dead patient. Speak up and ask questions!

◆ Learn all that you can about taking good care of yourself - body, mind and spirit.

◆ If all else fails --get a "retired" seeing eye dog!! And laugh and laugh and laugh.

THE END

Endnotes

[1] Writing Group for the Women's Health Initiative Investigators: Jacques E. Rossouw, Garnet L. Anderson, Ross L. Prentice, Andrea Z LaCroix, Charles Keeperberg, Fred Hutchinson, Marcia L, Stefanick, Rebecca D. Jackson, Shirely A. A. Beresford, Barbara V. Howard, Karen C. Johnson, Jane Morely Kotchen, Judith Ockene. Risks and Benefits of Estrogen Plus Progestin in Healthy Postmenopausal Women. *Journal of the American Medical Association,* 2002; 288 (3)

[2] Kolata, Gina, Menopause Without Pills: Rethinking Hot Flashes, *The New York Times,* November 10, 2002

[3] Ibid

[4] Postmenopausal Hormones: Where do we go from here? *Harvard Women's Health Watch,* 2003, 10 (5)pp3-4.

[5] Ibid

Jean Macpherson Duffy

About the Author:

Jean Macpherson Duffy is no stranger to controversy.

The first registered nurse elected to the California Legislature, she is known for her independence. Changing her political party while in office taught this feisty mother of five how to make tough decisions in her struggle for better health care.

Jean passed the nation's toughest drunk driving legislation and worked to form MADD (Mothers Against Drunk Driving). The Jean M. Duffy Award for Legislative Initiative in that field is awarded annually in many states.

Jean brings the same focus and determination to breast cancer treatment.

When elected she was Associate Professor of Nursing at the local university. Alzheimer's Disease and seniors rights are also priorities with this Stanford University graduate.

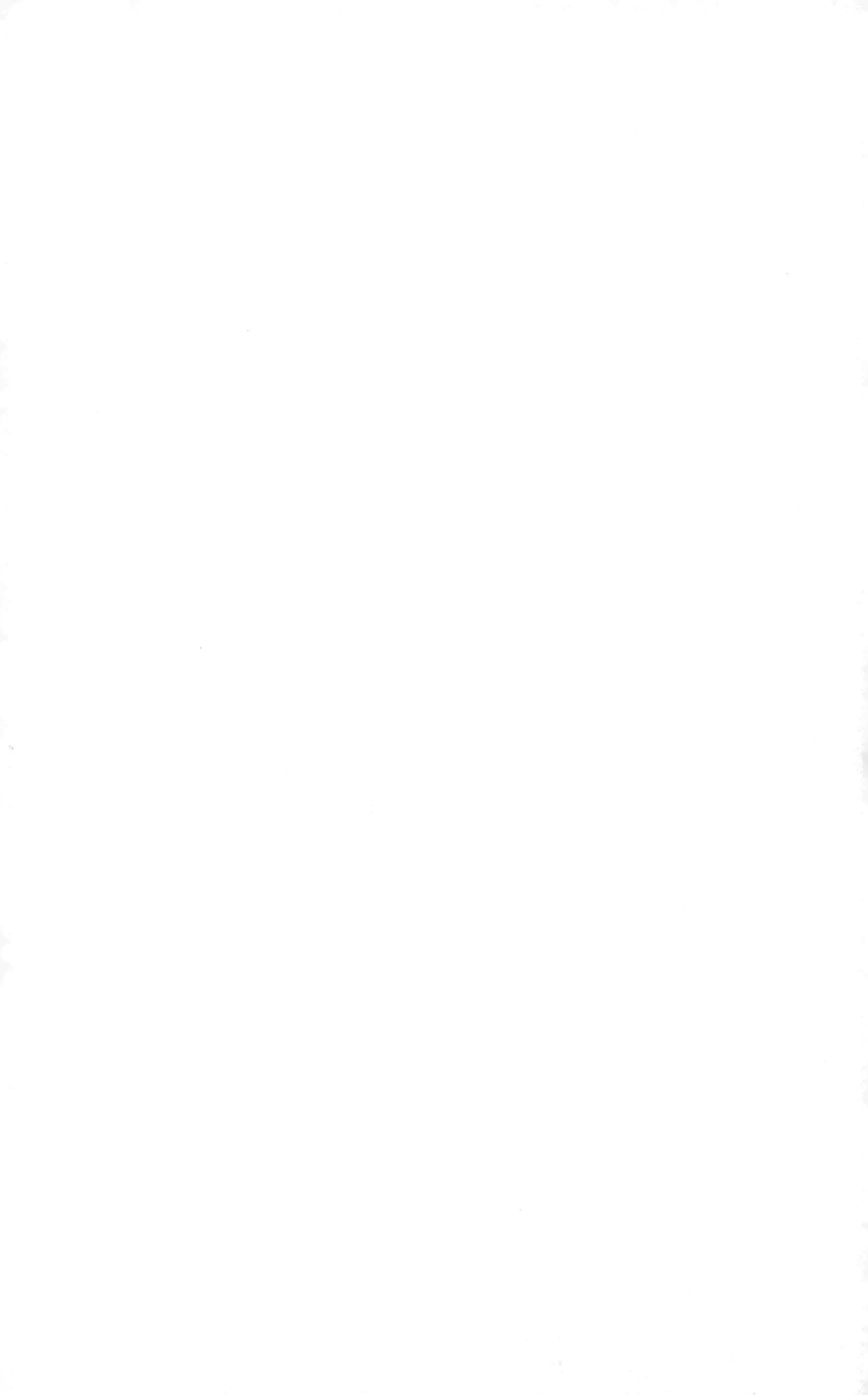